DIMENSIONS OF SCIENCE
Series Editor: Professor Jeff Thompson

HUMAN REPRODUCTION AND *in vitro* FERTILISATION

H. J. Leese

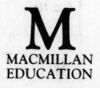

MACMILLAN
EDUCATION

First published 1988

Published by
MACMILLAN EDUCATION LTD
Houndmills, Basingstoke, Hampshire RG21 2XS
and London
Companies and representatives
throughout the world

Printed in Hong Kong

British Library Cataloguing in Publication Data
Leese, H. J. (Henry J)
    Human reproduction and in vitro
    fertilisation.
    1. Women. Ova. In vitro fertilisation.
    Social aspects
    I. Title   II. Series
    362.1'042

ISBN 0-333-45121-X

For Brenda, David and Matthew

Series Standing Order

If you would like to receive future titles in this series as they are published, you can make use of our standing order facility. To place a standing order please contact your bookseller or, in case of difficulty, write to us at the address below with your name and address and the name of the series. Please state with which title you wish to begin your standing order. (If you live outside the United Kingdom we may not have the rights for your area, in which case we will forward your order to the publisher concerned.)

Customer Services Department, Macmillan Distribution Ltd
Houndmills, Basingstoke, Hampshire, RG21 2XS, England.

Contents

Series Editor's Preface

This book is one in a Series designed to illustrate and explore a range of ways in which scientific knowledge is generated, and techniques are developed and applied. The volumes in this Series will certainly satisfy the needs of students at 'A' level and in first-year higher-education courses, although there is no intention to bridge any apparent gap in the transfer from secondary to tertiary stages. Indeed, the notion that a scientific education is both continuous and continuing is implicit in the approach which the authors have taken.

Working from a base of 'common core' 'A'-level knowledge and principles, each book demonstrates how that knowledge and those principles can be extended in academic terms, and also how they are applied in a variety of contexts which give relevance to the study of the subject. The subject matter is developed both in depth (in intellectual terms) and in breadth (in relevance). A significant feature is the way in which each text makes explicit some aspect of the fundamental processes of science, or shows science, and scientists, 'in action'. In some cases this is made clear by highlighting the methods used by scientists in, for example, employing a systematic approach to the collection of information, or the setting up of an experiment. In other cases the treatment traces a series of related steps in the scientific process, such as investigation, hypothesising, evaluating and problem-solving. The fact that there are many dimensions to the creation of knowledge and to its application by scientists and technologists is the title and consistent theme of all the books in the Series.

The authors are all authorities in the fields in which they have written, and share a common interest in the enjoyment of their work in science. We feel sure that something of that satisfaction will be imparted to their readers in the continuing study of the subject.

Preface

This book began as a lecture to the Annual Meeting of The Association for Science Education, in York in 1986. I thank Mary Waltham of Macmillan Education for suggesting I turn the lecture into a book, and for her encouragement and advice during its writing.

The book is an attempt to take one example of modern biology, *in vitro* fertilisation (IVF), and place it in its social context. In practice, this has meant describing the biology of IVF, the social aspects of the science surrounding it, the incidence and nature of infertility, the clinical procedures involved in IVF, the ethical issues raised and the response of Government. In other words, the book explores separately some of the multidisciplinary aspects of IVF. Since so much of the subject matter is open to a variety of interpretations, it has largely been left to readers to form their own overview of this fascinating topic.

While every effort has been made to present the latest information, this is a very fast-moving field, in which the state of the art changes rapidly. I hope readers will bear with the occasional fact or statement that has been overtaken by events.

I thank Drs John Biggers, Dave Gardner and Liz Lenton for their valuable comments on parts of the book and Michael Hooper for so skilfully drawing the diagrams. Ultimate responsibility for everything in the book is, of course, mine.

Finally I am indebted to Bob Edwards for introducing me to that wonder of nature, the early human embryo, and to my wife, for her constant support and quintessentially female viewpoint.

Acknowledgements

The author and publishers wish to thank the following who have kindly given permission for the use of copyright material.

The Benjamin/Cummings Publishing Company for illustrations based on *The World of the Cell* by Wayne M. Becker, pp. 491 and 620. Copyright © 1986.

The Controller of Her Majesty's Stationery Office for extracts from *Human Fertilisation and Embryology: A Framework for Legislation*, Cm. 259, DHSS.

Macdonald & Co. (Publishers) Ltd for a diagram based on *Infertility: A Sympathetic Approach* by Robert M. L. Winston, p. 159, Martin Dunitz.

Macmillan Magazines Ltd for extracts from 'Social Values and Research in Human Embryology' by Robert G. Edwards and David J. Sharpe, *Nature*, Vol. 231, 14.5.71 and 'Early Stages of Fertilization *in vitro* of Human Oocytes Matured *in vitro*' by R. G. Edwards, B. D. Bavister and P. C. Steptoe, *Nature*, Vol. 221, 15.2.69.

Sereno Laboratories Ltd for illustration based on 'In Vitro Fertilisation: Some Questions Answered', p. 7.

Every effort has been made to trace all the copyright holders but if any have been inadvertently overlooked the publishers will be pleased to make the necessary arrangement at the first opportunity.

List of Abbreviations

AID	Artificial Insemination by Donor
AIH	Artificial Insemination by Husband
FSH	Follicle Stimulating Hormone
GnRH	Gonadotrophin Releasing Hormone
HCG	Human Chorionic Gonadotrophin
HMG	Human Menopausal Gonadotrophin
IVF	*in vitro* Fertilisation
LH	Luteinising Hormone
LHRH	Gonadotrophin Releasing Hormone
MRC	Medical Research Council
RCOG	Royal College of Obstetricians and Gynaecologists
SLA	Statutory Licensing Authority
VLA	Voluntary Licensing Authority

1 The Biology of Human Fertilisation

Fertilisation is the union of the two gametes (the egg and the sperm) and takes place in the Fallopian tube or oviduct. While in the Fallopian tube, the fertilised egg divides to form a ball of cells, known as the *preimplantation embryo*, which then passes into the uterus or womb. Implantation begins on about the sixth day following fertilisation, and if all goes well, a baby will be born about 9 months later.

During *in vitro* fertilisation (literally, fertilisation in glass), the events which normally occur in the Fallopian tube (that is, *in vivo*) are by-passed. Eggs and sperm are brought together in a small culture dish and the resulting embryo is artificially replaced in the mother's uterus.

Before we can consider *in vitro* fertilisation or IVF as it is usually known, it is necessary to outline the biology of human fertilisation, and the events which precede and follow it, in order to indicate which processes need to be mimicked *in vitro*.

SPERM PRODUCTION (SPERMATOGENESIS)

Spermatozoa are manufactured in the testis in a hormonally controlled process known as spermatogenesis (figure 1.1). The cells from which the sperm are made are called *spermatogonia*. They are diploid cells with 46 chromosomes; 44 autosomes and two sex chromosomes, the X chromosome and the Y chromosome. During spermatogenesis, the spermatogonia are transformed via primary spermatocytes, secondary spermatocytes and spermatids into spermatozoa, the whole process taking about 10 weeks. Spermatogonia are replaced by cell division (mitosis) throughout life, with a slight increase in production at puberty.

Spermatozoa are haploid cells with 23 chromosomes, 22 autosomal plus an X chromosome or a Y chromosome. If a sperm bearing an X chromosome fertilises an egg, the baby will normally be female, whereas the product of the union of a Y sperm with an egg will normally be male. The process by which the chromosome number is halved is called *meiosis* and

1

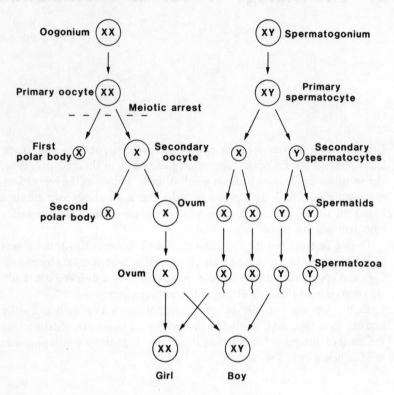

Figure 1.1 *Diagram of spermatogenesis and oogenesis*

it too occurs during egg formation. The adult chromosome number is thus restored at fertilisation.

Spermatogenesis will not take place at body temperature (37°C), the testes being held in the scrotum, outside the body cavity, at a temperature of about 34°C (figure 1.2). There are well documented cases of sterility in long distance lorry drivers wearing tight underwear in over-heated cabs, and in men taking excessively hot baths each day.

Sperm artificially removed from the testis are infertile and need to undergo further maturation in the vasa efferentia, the epididymis and the vas deferens. The epididymis is a coiled tubular structure, more than 20 feet in length in which the sperm are thought to spend up to 18 days. The most obvious difference between sperm removed from the testis and from the end of the epididymis is in motility. Testicular sperm are weakly

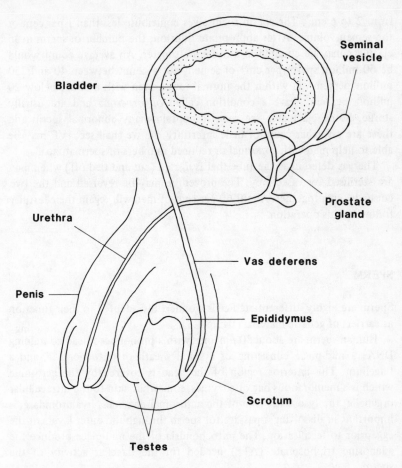

Figure 1.2 *Diagram of the male reproductive tract*

motile, whereas epididymal sperm, on exposure to an appropriate medium, exhibit a vigorous, progressive motion.

SEMEN

At ejaculation, sperm mainly from the epididymis, are expelled along the vas deferens and out through the penis, being joined as they go by copious secretions from the seminal vesicles and the prostate gland. The mixture of secretions (seminal plasma) and sperm is called *semen*. Its volume ranges

3

from 2 to 6 cm^3. The sperm themselves contribute less than 1 per cent of the semen volume. After appropriate dilution, the number of sperm in an ejaculate may be counted in a haemocytometer. An average count would be 60 million sperm per cm^3 of semen, but a count between 40 and 250 million per cm^3 is within the normal range. Men with a count below 20 million per cm^3 have a condition called *oligospermia* and are usually sterile. Some ejaculates are seen to contain many abnormal sperm and these are a further cause of male infertility. As we shall see, IVF may be able to help men with abnormal or reduced numbers of spermatozoa.

The vas deferens is the tube that is ligated (cut and tied off) when men are sterilised by vasectomy. The procedure may be reversed and the two cut ends sewn together. About 60 per cent of men will regain their fertility following this operation.

SPERM

Sperm are highly differentiated cells wonderfully adapted to their function as carriers of genetic material (figure 1.3).

Human sperm are about 50 μm long, with a pronounced head containing DNA, a mid-piece consisting of a spiral sheath of mitochondria, and a flagellum. The anterior region of the head is covered by the acrosome which is a membranous bag of enzymes, somewhat akin to the intracellular organelle, the lysosome. One of the acrosomal enzymes, hyaluronidase, is important in dissolving a passage for sperm through the outer layers of the egg prior to fertilisation. The mitochondria of the mid-piece produce the adenosine triphosphate (ATP) needed for the flagellar activity of the sperm.

Sperm are metabolically versatile. They can synthesise ATP by oxidising fats contained within them. Sperm can also oxidise pyruvic and lactic acids which are present in oviduct fluid at the site of fertilisation. Finally, they can oxidise sugars such as glucose, which is also present in the secretions of the female reproductive tract. This mitochondrial 'aerobic respiration' is highly efficient and can generate 38 molecules of ATP from the complete oxidation of a molecule of glucose.

It is curious to note that the characteristic sugar of semen is not glucose but fructose, produced largely by the seminal vesicles. However, sperm consume glucose faster than fructose, and glucose is added routinely, as are pyruvic and lactic acids, to the media used for IVF. Why the 'male' sugar should be fructose is a mystery. When the need arises, perhaps at high sperm densities in the vagina and cervix, sperm can metabolise sugars

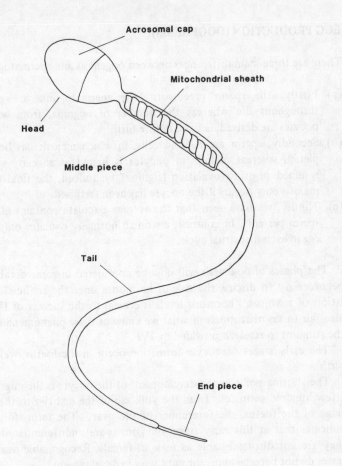

Figure 1.3 *Diagram of a human spermatozoon*

anaerobically, producing lactic acid. This is a less efficient process with a net yield of only two ATP molecules per molecule of glucose.

The ATP made in the mid-piece has to diffuse to the contractile elements in the tail. Theoretical calculations have shown that the tail is just the right length to ensure that sufficient ATP reaches the tip despite its being consumed *en route*.

EGG PRODUCTION (OOGENESIS)

There are three main differences between oogenesis and spermatogenesis:

(a) Firstly, the sperm precursors – the spermatogonia are produced throughout life whereas the number of oogonia, from which the oocytes are derived, is fixed before birth.
(b) Secondly, sperm are haploid cells, in which meiosis has been completed, whereas meiosis in oocytes is halted at an early stage and resumed prior to ovulation (figure 1.1). Indeed, the final phase of meiosis only occurs if the oocyte has been fertilised.
(c) Thirdly, we have seen that the average ejaculate contains 60 million sperm per cm^3. In contrast, a woman normally ovulates only a single egg in each menstrual cycle.

The phases of oogenesis will now be considered in some detail. It will be necessary to discuss the role of hormones since the artificial manipulation of a woman's hormone levels is crucial to the success of IVF. It is also fair to say that much of what we know of these phenomena is due to the stimulus to research provided by IVF.

The early stages of oocyte formation occur in the foetus, well before birth.

The starting point in the development of the oocyte is the migration of a few hundred germ cells from the yolk sac of the embryo to the genital ridge of the foetus, the forerunner of the ovary. The term 'forerunner' indicates that at this early stage, the gonads are undifferentiated, that is they are not distinguishable as male or female. Recognisable ovaries and testes do not become apparent until later in development.

The migration of germ cells begins around the third week of pregnancy. The numbers of these oogonia in the foetal ovary are increased by mitosis to about 7 million by the fourth or fifth month of gestation. Mitosis then ceases and the numbers of oogonia decline precipitously, mainly by a process of progressive wastage known as *atresia*, so that by birth, they now number about 2 million. Of these, one million are degenerate. By puberty, the number is reduced to approximately 40,000. Coincident with this decline before birth is the initiation of meiosis, at which point the oogonia are termed *primary oocytes*.

MEIOSIS

Meiosis may be thought of as two cellular divisions, with only one duplication of the chromosomes (figure 1.4).

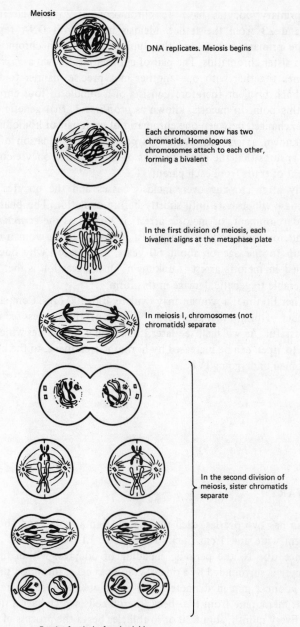

Meiosis

DNA replicates. Meiosis begins

Each chromosome now has two chromatids. Homologous chromosomes attach to each other, forming a bivalent

In the first division of meiosis, each bivalent aligns at the metaphase plate

In meiosis I, chromosomes (not chromatids) separate

In the second division of meiosis, sister chromatids separate

Result of meiosis: four haploid cells, each with half as many chromosomes as the original cell

Figure 1.4 *Diagram of meiosis*

The primary oocytes have 46 chromosomes; 23 derived from the mother and 23 from the father. Meiosis begins with DNA replication within the primary oocyte and the duplication of each chromosome to form two sister chromatids. The pair of chromatids, known as *homologues* now comes together with one another in a precise manner to form bivalents. Each bivalent therefore consists of a bundle of four chromatids. It is at this point in meiosis, known as *prophase 1*, that genetic material may be exchanged between one chromatid of each pair of homologues in a process known as *crossing over*. This possible recombination of genetic material ensures that the chromosomes of the resulting oocyte contain an assortment of traits from each parent.

Shortly after crossing over, meiosis ceases and the oocytes enter a resting phase which lasts until shortly before ovulation. This phase of suspended development, or meiotic arrest, is known as the *germinal vesicle stage*, and for some oocytes can persist for as long as a woman ovulates, that is up to the age of about 50 years. The reason why oocytes are maintained in meiotic arrest is unknown. One suggestion is that they are less vulnerable to genetic damage in this form.

Over her lifetime, a woman may ovulate 400–500 eggs. Compared with the number of primordial germ cells (7 million), this process seems excessively wasteful. As we shall see later, the number of oocytes which can be induced to ripen can be increased by hormone treatment, to the benefit of those women undergoing IVF.

THE OVARY

A woman has two ovaries, each the shape of an almond, and about 4 cm long, 2 cm wide and 1 cm thick. The surface of the ovary has a scarred appearance due to the periodic shedding of oocytes. Within the ovary, each oocyte is surrounded by a ring of granulosa cells, forming a primordial follicle, about 2 mm in diameter. The granulosa cells are separated by a basement membrane from the theca interna cells, which have a rich blood supply. Every month, about 20 or so follicles begin the process of development which culminates in ovulation, but only one usually reaches this end point. The remainder degenerate by atresia. How the chosen follicle is selected is a mystery.

8

FOLLICULAR DEVELOPMENT

As the follicle matures, the numbers of granulosa cells increase until five or six layers surround the oocyte (figure 1.5). Fluid then begins to appear in spaces among the cells and the spaces gradually coalesce to form a fluid-filled cavity, the antrum. The growth of the follicles is under the control of hormones called oestrogens. The initial reactions of oestrogen bio-synthesis are thought to occur in the theca cells, the final stages in the granulosa cells. The follicle continues to enlarge so that by the day of ovulation, it may be over 2 cm in diameter and contain up to 10 cm^3 of fluid. By now the oocyte is suspended in the follicular fluid by a small stalk of granulosa cells. The cells immediately surrounding the oocyte are known as *cumulus cells*, and these are shed, along with the oocyte, at ovulation.

As ovulation approaches, meiosis, which we will recall had been arrested at the germinal vesicle stage, resumes (figure 1.4). The homologous chromo-somes in the primary oocytes become arranged on the meiotic spindle, the first meiotic division takes place and the bivalents move apart. The division of the cytoplasm is unequal. One-half of the chromosomes remain in the main body of the oocyte, now known as a *secondary oocyte*, the other half migrate into a cytoplasmic bleb, which is subsequently pinched off to form the first polar body. Note that the sister chromatids still remain attached to one another at this first meiotic division, it is the homologues that separate. Thus, the secondary oocyte and the first polar body each contain the haploid number of duplicated chromosomes.

The second meitotic division follows almost immediately. The chromo-somes in the secondary oocyte become aligned on the second metaphase plate and meiosis is arrested for the second time. It is in this form that the oocytes are shed from the ovary into the Fallopian tube.

OVULATION

Ovulation occurs around the 14th day of the menstrual cycle. The mature follicle ruptures, and the oocyte with its surrounding cumulus cells and a small quantity of sticky follicular fluid is expelled. Following ovulation, the crater-like follicle fills with blood, and the remaining granulosa cells proliferate and transform the follicle into the corpus luteum, which secretes mainly the hormone progesterone. If pregnancy ensues, the corpus luteum (literally 'yellow body') remains active. Otherwise, it begins to degenerate after about 10 days, becoming a corpus albicans.

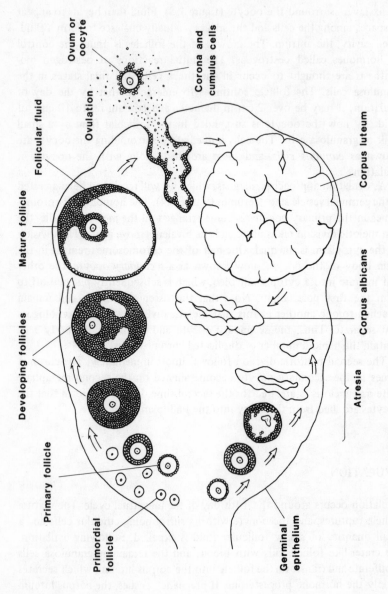

Figure 1.5 *Diagram of follicular development in the ovary*

Ovum or oocyte

Corona and cumulus cells

Follicular fluid

Ovulation

Corpus luteum

Mature follicle

Corpus albicans

Developing follicles

Atresia

Primary follicle

Primordial follicle

Germinal epithelium

A moment's thought illustrates the dilemma which this sequence of events poses for IVF. Once the egg has been released from the ovary, it is lost in the folds of the Fallopian tube and its recovery is virtually impossible. The egg has therefore to be collected from the ripe ovarian follicle: but when to collect it, and could more eggs be persuaded to ripen? The answers to these problems came from research on the hormonal control of oogenesis.

HORMONAL CONTROL

The endocrine control of female reproduction is complicated, and only a brief outline is given here (figure 1.6). Regulation is at three levels: the hypothalamus, the pituitary and the ovaries. The hypothalamus produces Gonadotrophin Releasing Hormone (GnRH) which stimulates the anterior pituitary to synthesise and secrete Follicle Stimulating Hormone (FSH) and Luteinising Hormone (LH). FSH stimulates the development of ovarian follicles and the production of oestrogen. Rising oestrogen levels stimulate a mid-cycle surge of LH which triggers ovulation and the formation of the corpus luteum. The ovarian hormones also induce rhythmical changes in the oviducts, uterus, cervix and vagina in preparation for a possible pregnancy. Needless to say, there are extensive feedback relationships between the various components of the endocrine system. As we shall see in chapter 4, the ability to detect the rise in LH has solved the problem of when to collect the egg for IVF. Furthermore, the administration of a mixture of FSH and LH stimulates follicular maturation and the production of more than one oocyte.

PREDICTION OF OVULATION

It is appropriate at this point to mention the simplest, if not the most reliable method by which a woman can determine whether ovulation is imminent. She may want to do this to know when she is most likely to be fertile.

Progesterone is a mildly thermogenic hormone, that is it increases the basal metabolic rate, and hence the body temperature. Immediately after ovulation, the temperature rises by about $0.2^{\circ}C$ (or $0.4^{\circ}F$), whereas prior to ovulation it usually drops (figure 1.7).

It is best to take the temperature on waking and to record the value on a chart. Since the body temperature varies from day to day, the chart can

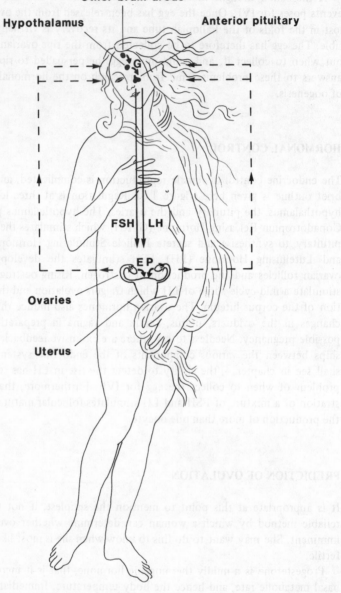

Figure 1.6 *Simplified diagram of the hormonal control of reproduction in the woman. (After Botticelli, The Birth of Venus) [G (GnRH); E (oestrogen); P (progesterone)]*

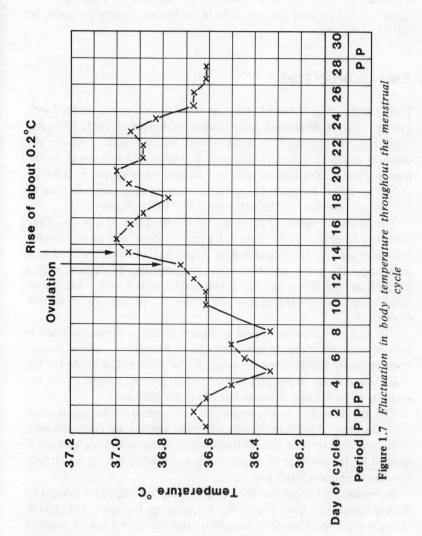

Figure 1.7 *Fluctuation in body temperature throughout the menstrual cycle*

13

only really be interpreted at the end of the menstrual cycle when it is easier to average out the fluctuations.

Precise timing of intercourse is unnecessary for most couples wishing to conceive, because human sperm are relatively long-lived in the female reproductive tract, but on the basis of the temperature chart shown in figure 1.7, the optimal time would be in the hours following ovulation, on day 13 of the cycle.

THE FALLOPIAN TUBE

The Fallopian tube is named after Gabriele Fallopius who is credited with the first correct description of the organ, in Venice in 1561. The other name for the Fallopian tube is the oviduct, which is used to refer to the organ in mammals generally. The term Fallopian tube is reserved for the human. Doctors also tend to refer to Fallopian tubes as 'uterine tubes' or simply as 'tubes'. Defective Fallopian tubes are the most common cause of infertility in women, and the main reason why IVF was developed.

The tubes are about 12 cm long and the thickness of a pencil. They consist of an outer muscular coat with a mucous lining, and may be divided into three regions: the *infundibulum*, shaped like a funnel, and lined with long finger-like folds, called fimbriae; the *ampulla*, thin-walled, with a highly branched lining; and the *isthmus*, thick-walled with a less convoluted lining. The isthmus leads to the uterus, via the utero–tubal junction (figure 1.8).

The lining or mucosa, known in clinical circles as the *endosalpinx*, is covered with two types of cells – ciliated and secretory – whose proportions gradually change along the length of the oviduct. The top end of the ampulla has about 70 per cent ciliated and 30 per cent secretory cells, the opposite being the case at the uterine end of the isthmus.

The infundibulum is responsible for the capture of the egg released from the ovary. The fimbriae, which like the ampulla are richly endowed with cilia, tend to close around the ovary at ovulation and egg 'pick-up' is assisted by the presence of cumulus cells surrounding the egg which help the cilia to obtain a better grip.

Movement of the egg–cumulus complex along the ampulla is thought to depend largely on ciliary action. For example, egg transport is blocked in the rabbit if a short length of ampulla is surgically turned around, whereas this is not the case in the isthmus, where muscular contractions are thought to be more important in transporting the resulting embryo.

Human eggs are thought to take up to 24 hours to traverse the ampulla. Fertilisation takes place just above the junction of the ampulla with the

14

isthmus. Nutrients for the egg, sperm and for the embryo while it resides in the tube are provided by oviduct fluid, a complex watery secretion containing salts, the energy sources glucose, pyruvic acid and lactic acid, amino acids and other small and large molecules. Knowledge of the composition of oviduct fluid was important in devising the media used for *in vitro* fertilisation and embryo culture.

THE UTERUS

The human uterus is a pear-shaped organ, about 7 cm long and 5 cm at its widest point. In cross-section, it is seen to consist of two main layers: an outer myometrium composed of smooth muscle and an inner endometrium in turn divided into two parts. Bordering the lumen of the uterus is a single layer of epithelial cells which also form the lining of invaginations known as 'uterine glands'. The rest of the endometrium is termed the stroma.

In women and other female primates, much of the endometrium is lost at menstruation, as part of a cycle of uterine changes (figure 1.9). If the onset of menstruation is taken as day 1, the menstrual phase lasts 4–5 days. Under the influence of FSH, a new crop of follicles begins to ripen in the ovary and the oestrogens they produce stimulate the growth of the uterine endometrium. This is the preovulatory or follicular phase, which lasts about 10 days. The rise in oestrogen triggers the burst of LH secretion which brings about ovulation.

The postovulatory or luteal phase lasts about 14 days. It is also termed the *progestational phase* because of the increasing amounts of progesterone secreted by the corpus luteum in anticipation of the possible arrival of an embryo. The endometrium continues to proliferate, accumulate large amounts of the energy reserve glycogen, and develop a copious blood supply.

If pregnancy does not occur, the corpus luteum begins to degenerate, progesterone and oestrogen levels fall, the blood vessels in the uterus constrict leading to ischaemia (lack of oxygen) in the endometrium and the onset of menstruation.

THE PASSAGE OF SPERM THROUGH THE FEMALE TRACT

Out of an average of 350 million sperm deposited in the vagina at intercourse, only a few hundred are thought to reach the site of fertilisation in the Fallopian tube. Various physical and physiological barriers await

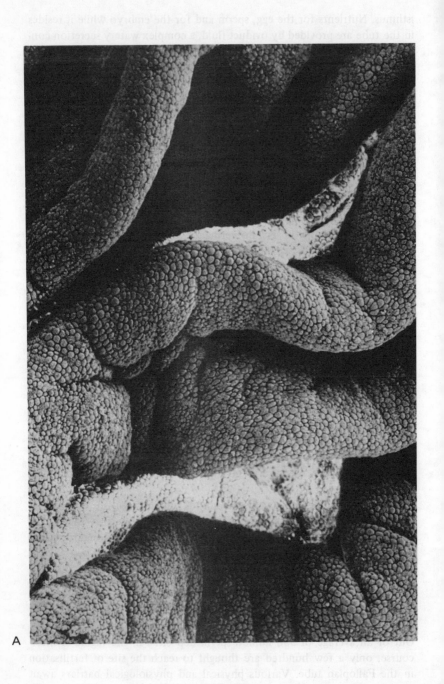

A

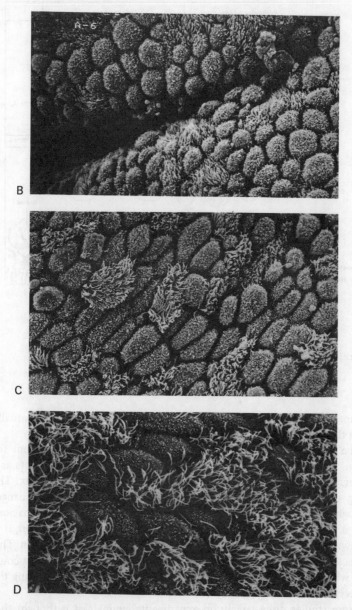

Figure 1.8 *Scanning electron micrographs of the surface lining of the Fallopian tube, at increasing magnification (A–D). Note the extensive folding and the two types of cells (ciliated and secretory) which cover the surface. (Photographs by courtesy of Peter G. Humpherson)*

17

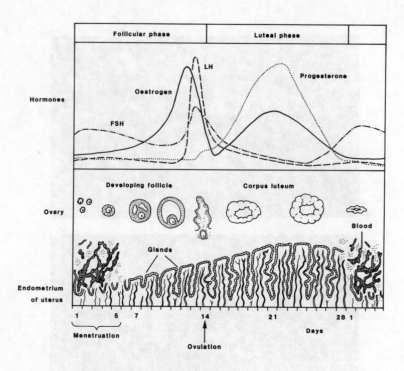

Figure 1.9 *The menstrual cycle*

the sperm on their journey (figure 1.10). The few sperm that eventually reach the ampulla are probably a selected, more fertile, population.

The vagina, with a pH of around 5.7, is a hostile environment for sperm, even though semen, with a pH of between 7.2 and 7.8, acts as a buffer. To reach the uterus, the sperm have to negotiate the cervix. The lining of the cervix is covered with mucus, whose composition changes throughout the menstrual cycle. After ovulation it is thick and tenacious with a high content of a protein called mucin, but before ovulation, it is very watery, less viscous and offers a favourable passage to the sperm. This characteristic of cervical mucus is the basis of the so-called post-coital test, which has been used for over 100 years as an aid to discovering the cause(s) of infertility (page 41).

From studies done largely on experimental animals, it is thought that the numbers of sperm reaching the uterus is rather small — maybe only 1 per cent of the number in the ejaculate, and that the cervix may act as a

18

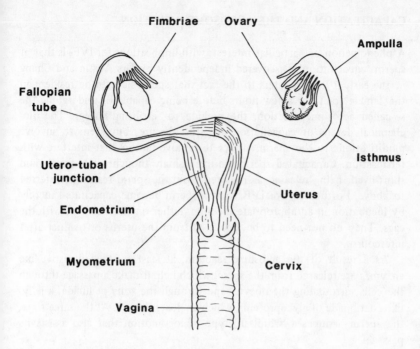

Figure 1.10 *Diagram of the female reproductive tract*

'reservoir', releasing waves of sperm, as required, into the uterus. Further sperm reservoirs exist at the utero-tubal junction and the ampullary-isthmus junction in the Fallopian tube. Since intercourse cannot be timed to anticipate ovulation exactly, the presence of these reservoirs may help to maximise the chances of sperm being present in the Fallopian tube when the egg finally arrives. They may also explain why sperm can remain fertile for so long within the woman; up to 5 days according to some, and one reason why the 'safe period' method of contraception is so unreliable.

While one might imagine intuitively that sperm swim under their own power from the site of insemination to that of fertilisation, this is not the case. Maximum swimming rates of about 0.1 mm/second are unable to account for the fact that sperm have been found in human Fallopian tubes within 15 minutes of coitus. This indicates that sperm transport must largely be a function of the contractile activity of the female tract. Intrinsic sperm motility is probably important only in traversing the cervical mucus, the utero-tubal junction and the outer vestments of the egg.

19

CAPACITATION AND THE ACROSOME REACTION

A phenomenon of particular interest, with implications for IVF, is that of sperm 'capacitation'. Discovered independently by Drs Austin and Chang in the early 1950s, it refers to the fact that sperm have to be resident in the female tract for a few hours before being capable of undergoing the so-called acrosome reaction, the prelude to fertilising an egg. The biochemical details of capacitation are still obscure, but seem to involve modifications to the sperm surface to remove factors that interfere with fertilisation. Capacitated sperm are increasingly thought of as fragile and short-lived, being released as required from the sperm reservoirs referred to above. Fortunately for IVF, human sperm become capacitated merely by incubation in an appropriate medium, either on their own or with the eggs. They do not need to be recovered from the uterus or oviduct after intercourse.

As a result of the acrosome reaction, at least a dozen digestive-like enzymes are released from the sperm which help it make a passage through the cells surrounding the oocyte, and through the zona pellucida, a jelly-like coat, made of glycoproteins, which encloses the egg. At the same time, the sperm assumes a 'whiplash' type of locomotion that also assists its passage.

FERTILISATION

When a sperm and the oocyte come into contact, the mid-region of the sperm head fuses with the outer membrane of the oocyte and the sperm enters the oocyte. Within 3 hours, the oocyte has completed its second meiotic division, in which the sister chromatids separate with the formation of the second polar body. After 6 hours, the haploid mass of chromosomes has been transformed into the female pronucleus, which over the next 12 hours migrates towards the male pronucleus, derived from the original sperm nucleus. The two pronuclei fuse and the first cell division takes place, about 24-28 hours after sperm penetration. The coming together of the gametic chromosomes is called *syngamy*.

After one sperm has entered the oocyte, a series of events is put in motion to prevent the entry of further sperm. This block to polyspermy has been extensively characterised in the eggs of the sea urchin and other invertebrates, but is less well understood in the mammal. A feature of IVF is the high incidence of embryos with three pronuclei, (triploidy), which probably arise from the entry of two sperms, suggesting that the block to polyspermy is less effective *in vitro*. Such embryos, although genetically abnormal, cleave normally for two or three days before degenerating.

THE DEVELOPMENT OF THE PREIMPLANTATION EMBRYO

The fertilised human ovum, or zygote, is about 120 μm (0.12 mm) in diameter, which is a very large cell by mammalian standards. It remains at this size for the next 2 or 3 days while dividing repeatedly to form a ball of progressively smaller, adult-sized cells (figures 1.11 and 1.12). The first 24 hours following fertilisation is probably spent in the ampulla of the Fallopian tube, the 2-cell, 4-cell, and 8–16 cell preimplantation stages in the isthmus. The embryo is thought to leave the Fallopian tube and enter the uterus on the third day following fertilisation by which time it has reached the morula stage of development. In other words, the first 3 or so days of life are spent in the Fallopian tube and not the uterus as is supposed by many. The morula, which looks like a blackberry, marks a key point in early differentiation in that the cells comprising it have become tightly opposed, with a greater proportion of their surfaces in contact. This is a prelude to the appearance of a cavity or blastocoel within the embryo, and the formation of the blastocyst on day 4. Prior to the formation of the morula, the embryo is somewhat quiescent in a metabolic sense. It derives its energy from the oxidation of pyruvic acid, but does so at a relatively slow rate and is not particularly active in protein synthesis. During this early preimplantation phase, its activities are controlled to a large extent by messenger RNA from the original oocyte. The new embryonic genetic material does not take over complete control of events until the blastocyst stage, when rates of protein synthesis are similar to adult cells. This molecular information is sometimes mentioned in debates on the question: 'when does human life begin?'

By day 5, the human blastocyst is composed of over 100 cells, about 90 of which encircle the blastocoel as the trophectoderm, the remainder being clustered together to form the inner cell mass. The embryo proper is ultimately derived from some of the cells of the inner cell mass. The extra-embryonic structures, such as the placenta, are derived from the trophectoderm and the other cells of the inner cell mass. This information of cell lineage is also brought into debates on the ethics of IVF as we shall see in chapter 6. The blastocyst remains unattached in the uterine lumen until about the sixth day following fertilisation when it begins to implant.

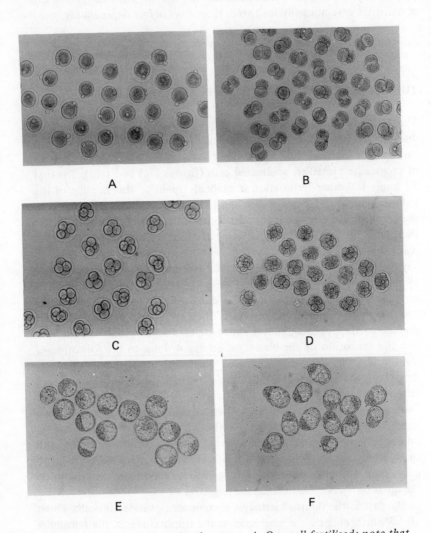

Figure 1.11 *Mouse embryo development: A. One-cell fertilised: note that in most cases, one of the polar bodies has been lost; B. 2-cell embryos; C. 4-cell embryos; D. 8-cell embryos and early morulae; E. Blastocysts: note the blastocoel cavity, and collection of cells which comprise the inner cell mass; F. Blastocysts which have hatched from the zona pellucida. (Photographs by courtesy of Dr David Gardner and Amanda Gott)*

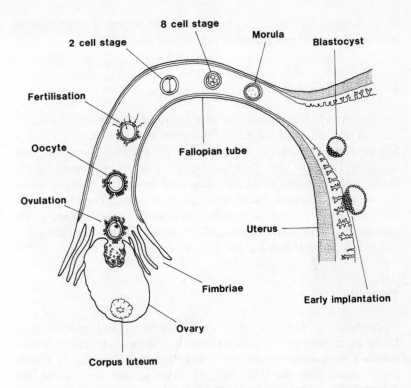

Figure 1.12 *Development of early human embryos from ovulation to implantation*

IMPLANTATION

Begore it can implant, the blastocyst has to 'hatch' from the zona pellucida. Once the zona has been lost, on about day 6, the embryo can penetrate the epithelium of the endometrium and begin to bed down in the stroma. Implantation takes about a week. It is day 10-11 before the embryo is completely buried and day 13-14 before implantation can be said to have been completed.

For implantation to be successful, it is obvious that the normal menstrual cycle must be interrupted so as to prevent menstruation and the loss of the embryo. The likely way in which this is achieved in the mother is by the production of the hormone Human Chorionic Gonadotrophin (HCG) by the blastocyst. The HCG acts as a signal to maintain the corpus luteum, which releases large amounts of oestrogen and progesterone. After about 6 weeks, this function is taken over by the placenta. The presence of HCG in the urine is the basis of a laboratory test of pregnancy which may be used in the second week following conception (page 50).

ECTOPIC PREGNANCY

For reasons which are not well understood, implantation may sometimes occur at sites other than the uterus. This is referred to as ectopic pregnancy and seems only to occur in the human species. The most common ectopic site is the Fallopian tube. Such 'tubal pregnancies' are life-threatening and are terminated as soon as they are diagnosed. In such an abortion, one of the woman's Fallopian tubes is therefore removed. The incidence of ectopic pregnancy in normal reproduction is about 3 per thousand but this rises to 20 per thousand following IVF, indeed the first 'test-tube baby' was an ectopic pregnancy and had to be aborted.

TWINNING

Non-identical or 'dizygotic' twins result from the fertilisation of two eggs. Identical, 'monozygotic' twins are formed when a single embryo divides into two. Such division can occur at any stage up to about day 15 following fertilisation. In the U.K., dizygotic twins account for about 9, and monozygotic about 3, of every 1000 births.

EMBRYONIC LOSSES

Of 100 embryos conceived *in vivo*, perhaps 50-55 per cent are lost prior to and during implantation. A further 10 per cent may miscarry, most frequently at 7-10 weeks gestation. In other words, it is likely that only 1 in 3 fertilised eggs will be successfully carried to term. We are ignorant of the reasons for this high natural rate of abortion, but it is known that many embryos are genetically abnormal.

CONCLUSION

This account of human fertilisation and the events surrounding it enables us to identify the steps which need to be mimicked to make IVF a reality.

We can list them:

(1) increasing the number of ripe ovarian follicles;
(2) collecting eggs from the ovary and ensuring their survival *in vitro*;
(3) collecting sperm and ensuring their survival and maturation *in vitro*;
(4) carrying out fertilisation *in vitro*;
(5) culturing preimplantation human embryos;
(6) replacing preimplantation human embryos in the uterus.

The way in which these steps are carried out in clinical practice is described in chapter 4.

2   IVF and the Nature of Science

As an alternative to a conventional historical account of the scientific discoveries which led to the birth of the first test-tube baby in 1978, this chapter attempts to capture the spirit of the *Dimensions of Science* series by using the topic of IVF to illustrate the nature of "science" and scientists, 'in action'." This is done by listing twelve propositions which relate to the way science operates and using examples drawn from the history and current practice of IVF in an attempt to justify them. It should be emphasised that what follows is a personal account and while it is likely that the majority of scientists would agree with these propositions, there are undoubtedly some who would not, or would take issue with the way they have been justified here.

The twelve propositions are shown in Box 2.1.

Box 2.1

(1) Scientific discoveries build on previous scientific discoveries and their basis is frequently laid down by scientists in different branches of science.

(2) The outcome of scientific experiments cannot be known in advance.

(3) Many discoveries turn out to have a significance far-removed from the problem that they were designed to investigate.

(4) There are traps and pitfalls awaiting the scientist.

(5) Science has its own momentum but also responds to pressures from society.

(6) The social climate can influence the conduct of scientific research.

(7) Scientific research costs money.

(8) Scientists are human.

(9) Science provides benefits and problems for society.

(10) Science cannot provide solutions to all problems.

(11) Scientists should have no more say in solving society's problems than anyone else.

(12) It is a sterile society which says: 'We know enough, why search for more?'

---

(1) Scientific discoveries build on previous scientific discoveries and their basis is frequently laid down by scientists in different branches of science.

The first test-tube baby did not come as a bolt from the blue. The ideas and techniques behind it had long histories. Table 2.1 shows just some of the key events involved. The scientists have included anatomists, embryologists, microscopists, geneticists, doctors and vets. In other words, IVF has had many dimensions and many contributors.

(2) The outcome of scientific experiments cannot be known in advance.

This is an obvious statement, since if the outcome of an experiment were known, there would be no need to do the experiment. In practice, of course, scientists have some *expectation* of what the outcome of an experi-

27

Table 2.1 Some major events and findings in the history of IVF

Aristotle (384–322 BC) writes the first account of embryology

1561	Fallopius gives first correct anatomical description of Fallopian tube
1677	Discovery of mammalian spermatozoa by A. van Leeuwenhoek
1797	Recovery of embryos from rabbit Fallopian tube by W. C. Cruikshank
1827	Identification of an egg in a mammalian ovarian follicle by C. E. von Baer
1875– 1878	Understanding that fertilisation requires the fusion of one sperm with one egg by Hertwig (in the sea urchin), Van Beneden (in the rabbit) and Fol (in the starfish)
1890	First embryo transfer (in the rabbit) by W. Heape
1912	First culture of mammalian embryos by A. Brachet
1930	First experiments on IVF (in rabbits) by G. Pincus
1932	Publication of *Brave New World* by A. Huxley
1944	First attempt at IVF using human oocytes by J. Rock and M. F. Menkin
1949	Development of culture medium in which 8-cell mouse eggs developed to blastocysts by J. Hammond Jr
1951	Capacitation of sperm described independently by M. C. Chang and C. R. Austin
1958	Transfer of cultured mouse blastocysts to the uterus of another female followed by birth of live young (A. McLaren and J. D. Biggers)
1959	Unequivocal demonstration of IVF in the rabbit by M. C. Chang
1969	Demonstration of human oocyte fertilisation *in vitro* by R. G. Edwards, B. D. Bavister and P. C. Steptoe
1972	Successful freezing of mammalian embryos (mouse) described independently by I. Wilmut and D. G. Whittingham
1976	First human pregnancy (ectopic) after IVF and embryo transfer (P. C. Steptoe and R. G. Edwards)
1978	Birth of first child following IVF and embryo transfer (P. C. Steptoe and R. G. Edwards)
1983	U.K. government sets up Committee of Enquiry into Human Fertilisation

ment will be – they could not have planned it otherwise – but often the outcome is quite different from that expected. Furthermore, the anticipated result may be interpreted in different ways by other scientists, either at that time or subsequently. This again, is not surprising, since scientists frame their experiments in terms of some idea that they wish to investigate, and their interpretation of the results of an experiment tends to be loaded in terms of this idea. It often needs a different perspective, brought by a different scientist, to see the wider significance.

An example of this is provided by some of the work of the distinguished English scientist, Walter Heape, carried out towards the end of the last century. Heape is generally regarded as one of the founding fathers of reproductive biology and was a versatile scientist. In addition to the work to be described, he discovered the oestrous cycle, and invented a high-speed camera! Working in Cambridge, Heape set out

"to determine in the first place, what effect, if any, a uterine foster-mother would have upon her foster children and whether or not the presence and development of foreign ova in the uterus of a mother would affect the offspring of that mother born at the same time."

He described what he did:

"On the 27th April, 1890, two ova were obtained from an Angora doe rabbit which had been fertilised by an Angora buck thirty-two hours previously; the ova were undergoing segmentation, being divided into four segments. The ova were immediately transferred into the upper end of the fallopian tube of a Belgian doe rabbit which had been fertilised three hours before by a buck of the same breed as herself . . .

In due course this Belgian doe gave birth to six young – four of these resembled herself and her mate, while two of them were undoubted Angoras. The Angora young were characterised by the possession of long silky hair peculiar to the breed, and were total albinos, like their Angora parents."

So far as Heape was concerned, the result of his experiment was negative! – in that the uterus of the foster-mother had *not* affected the offspring which had been placed there artificially. However, inadvertently, Heape had discovered how to remove a preimplantation embryo from one animal and transfer it into the uterus of another of the same species, with the production of live young.

So, in addition to (2) we can add

(3) Many discoveries turn out to have a significance far-removed from the problem that they were designed to investigate.

We can pursue this line of thought and consider proposition (4).

(4) There are traps and pitfalls awaiting the scientist.

A number of biologists in the 1930s and 1940s claimed to have fertilised rabbit eggs *in vitro*. Following IVF, the zygotes were observed in culture and seen to divide in the manner of an early embryo. There was a pitfall to this interpretation, which was recognised by two of the scientists involved, Pincus and Enzmann. (Pincus is best known for his work on the development of the contraceptive pill.) The pitfall is the phenomenon of parthenogenesis whereby *unfertilised* eggs can undergo a few divisions spontaneously. In the words of Pincus:

> "to what extent therefore, the development observed in the ova in these experiments may be attributable to fertilisation, it is impossible to say."

Pincus and Enzmann, in recognising this pitfall, realised the way round it was to transplant the supposedly fertilised eggs into a recipient rabbit as had first been done by Heape in 1890. When this was done, they found that rabbits were born whose coat colour matched that expected of the transferred embryos, and felt confident enough in 1934 to say that:

> "we believe that this is the first certain demonstration that mammalian eggs can be fertilised *in vitro*."

Others were sceptical however, and felt that Pincus and Enzmann had not recognised a further pitfall — that the eggs which were transferred may have carried with them spermatozoa still attached, and that fertilisation then took place in the recipient uterus, that is *in vivo*. This was a distinct possibility since the supposedly fertilised eggs were only allowed about 30 minutes *in vitro* before being transferred.

These equivocal results were not resolved until 1959, when M.C. Chang showed conclusively that rabbit ova could be fertilised *in vitro*. The key feature of Chang's work was that fertilised ova were allowed to cleave normally to the 4-cell stage in culture, before being transferred, by which time the sperm used for the IVF would not have been viable.

Similar disagreements, justified at the time, attended the reports by R. G. Edwards and colleagues in 1969, of the fertilisation of human ova *in vitro*. The obvious proof of the phenomenon, i.e. the birth of a baby following IVF had to wait until 1978!

Pitfalls should not be thought of in a negative sense, as detracting from the advancement of scientific knowledge. On the contrary, they are fundamental to it, and illustrate the way one learns from one's mistakes. They also reflect the need for scientists to be critical and sceptical about each other's work. This scrutiny takes place mainly in the scientific literature, but also at scientific meetings and informally as scientists talk to and about each other. It is known as 'peer review' in that what one does is judged by one's fellow scientists. Peer review is absolutely central to the practice of science. It is the way in which 'quality control' is achieved. Scientists know that sooner or later they will have to submit their work for review, and that it will be found to be good, bad, indifferent or whatever. If they have cheated, it is likely they will be found out. Peer review is an imperfect mechanism, as imperfect as the human beings who administer it, but it is the best guarantee we have of ensuring that science remains open, honest, accessible, non-secretive and of high quality. Sadly, science subjected to such open scrutiny is very much in the minority in the world today since about three-quarters of global expenditure on science is for military purposes, where open disclosure is obviously not allowed. This digression however, leads us to consider what forces drive science generally and to proposition (5).

(5) Science has its own momentum but also responds to pressures from society.

Most of the early pioneers listed in table 2.1 would have been driven by sheer curiosity to discover more about nature. Indeed some would say that the pursuit of knowledge in an unfettered but responsible manner is one of the hallmarks of a civilised society. As we approach the present time, a second motive assumes increasing importance; to apply knowledge about science, including reproduction, to the service of man. There are many areas in which such knowledge has been, and is being applied. They include Artificial Insemination and embryo transfer in animal breeding, the preservation of the embryos of threatened species, the development of contraceptives and the treatment of infertility.

As new applications have emerged, new industries have come into being, manufacturing fertility hormones, kits to measure them, embryo culture equipment, surgical apparatus, special refrigerators for freezing embryos etc. A market will surely emerge for techniques used to diagnose genetic diseases. Some view these developments as undesirable. They see reproductive technologies as taking over people's, particularly women's, lives. Others see Aldous Huxley's fantasy *Brave New World* as coming to fruition with 'glass wombs' and 'embryo farms'. Others, including myself, see them on balance as welcome advances which enhance the quality of people's lives. Of course, there need to be safeguards to ensure that the human condition is not debased, and these are dealt with in chapter 6.

Returning to proposition (5), it is notoriously difficult to untangle the extent to which a given scientific development has been 'pushed' by basic, curiosity-orientated research or been 'pulled' by pressure from society. For example, Steptoe and Edwards in their book *A Matter of Life*, repeatedly referred to their great desire to help the infertile, but at the same time, they made major discoveries of a fundamental nature. It is undoubtedly the case that the current pull to research on human embryos is coming from the clinical need to increase the success of IVF procedures, which in turn, is being pulled by the enormous demand for infertility treatment, and from the need to develop methods to diagnose genetic diseases in early embryos. However, in the process of developing these procedures, much will be learned about the basic biology of early human development.

The 'pull' to science from society does not necessarily mean that the science required is, or can be, carried out immediately. An editorial in the *New England Journal of Medicine*, in 1937, describes the possibility of treating women with blocked Fallopian tubes by IVF, some 41 years before the first test-tube baby was born!

Another example of the possibility of the application of science anticipating the science itself is given in an article by Dr John Biggers and Dr Anne McLaren, written in 1958, in which they pointed to the many thousands of immature eggs in the ovary of a cow, which, if they could be matured and fertilised *in vitro* and transferred to the uterus, would give rise to many times the average of four calves born during a cow's lifetime. Research directed to this problem is, in fact, being very actively pursued at the present time.

This section can be summarised by saying that the way science is driven is complicated, but may be simplified to:

$$\text{Science} \longleftrightarrow \text{Society}$$

The significance is in the two-way arrow, that is science can generate knowledge of interest to society, and society can influence the problems it wishes science to investigate. This leads naturally to proposition (6).

(6) The social climate can influence the conduct of scientific research.

Two examples in support of this proposition may be cited, one ancient, the other modern.

It will be recalled that Walter Heape was interested in whether the mother carrying an embryo which was not her own could influence the characteristics of the subsequent offspring. This interest reflected a view widely held in cattle breeding circles at the time (1890) that the progeny of one mating could be influenced by a male that had previously mated with their mother. This theory was known as telegony, and had influenced Heape's thinking and the planning and interpretation of his experiments.

Although Steptoe and Edwards were opposed by much of the medical and scientific establishment, it can be said that the public at large were ready to accept 'test-tube babies'. Following the austerity of the 1940s and the economic recovery of the 1950s, the 1960s and early 1970s were times when social attitudes became more liberal; abortion and human reproduction were freely discussed. As women gained a greater say in society and became less dominated by men, the discussion of infertility was no longer taboo and the science to alleviate it welcomed. There are differences between different countries in these matters particularly over their attitudes to research on human embryos. These national differences defy easy analysis. Surprisingly, such research seems to be more acceptable in Catholic southern Europe than in the Protestant north, with the U.K. an exception. Perhaps more surprising has been the restriction of government support for research related to human IVF in the U.S.A. This restriction has not hindered the setting up of private IVF clinics in the U.S.A., where there are now more than anywhere else. This leads us conveniently to the proposition which sooner or later has to be faced:

(7) Scientific research costs money.

The development of IVF and present research in this area has cost comparatively little. Most of the costs are the salaries of the research workers involved; laboratory costs being modest in comparison. This is the case for most biological research and contrasts with parts of the physical sciences, where equipment costs for particle accelerators and radio astronomy, for example, are enormous by comparison. In pioneering the technique of IVF, Steptoe and Edwards worked on a shoestring budget. Most of the investment was in terms of their time, that of the ancillary hospital and laboratory staff, and of the volunteer patients involved in the early days of IVF.

The Medical Research Council (MRC), the largest single body which funds medical research in the U.K., turned down their requests for money as did the various Secretaries of State in the DHSS at the time. They felt the work was too speculative. There *is* now some sponsorship of research into IVF by the MRC with increasing support coming from the commercial companies involved, particularly those who manufacture the hormones used to stimulate the production of ova. The research itself is carried out in IVF clinics or in university or related departments with which they are associated. As we shall see in chapter 6, there are voluntary controls on the type of research which may be carried out.

The costs of IVF treatment as opposed to research are considered in chapter 4.

(8) Scientists are human.

It may seem strange to make this statement. It is meant to correct the false impression that scientists are white-coated creatures, devoid of feelings and lacking humanity and morals. This false image partly derives from the way in which scientists describe their work, which *is* in very sober, rational, logical, impersonal language. For a good recent account of why this is so, the reader could consult Barnes' book *About Science*.

However, the way the results of science are expressed should not be confused with the processes by which it is obtained. In fact, scientists are just like anyone else, with the same human strengths, failings and emotions. While scientists rarely betray their feelings in the scientific literature, they do so all the time in general conversation and elsewhere.

As examples of these two worlds which scientists inhabit, consider the fundamental paper by Edwards, Bavister and Steptoe, published in 1969, in the world's leading scientific journal *Nature*. It says, in characteristically dead-pan style:

> "Human oocytes have been matured and fertilised by spermatozoa *in vitro*. There may be certain clinical and scientific uses for human eggs fertilised by this procedure."

By contrast, the comment by Edwards on some scientific data obtained in collaborative work between his laboratory and the Department of Biology at York University is shown in figure 2.1. It describes his very human feelings on realising that a single human embryo could have its metabolism studied without harming it, and that it could then go on to divide normally.

Propositions (9), (10) and (11):

(9) Science provides benefits and problems for society.
(10) Science cannot provide solutions to all problems.
(11) Scientists should have no more say in solving society's problems than anyone else.

IVF provides a classic example of the way in which science benefits people but at the same time poses dilemmas for society.

The obvious benefit is the alleviation of human infertility, but there are other likely benefits including the possibility of improved or new contra-

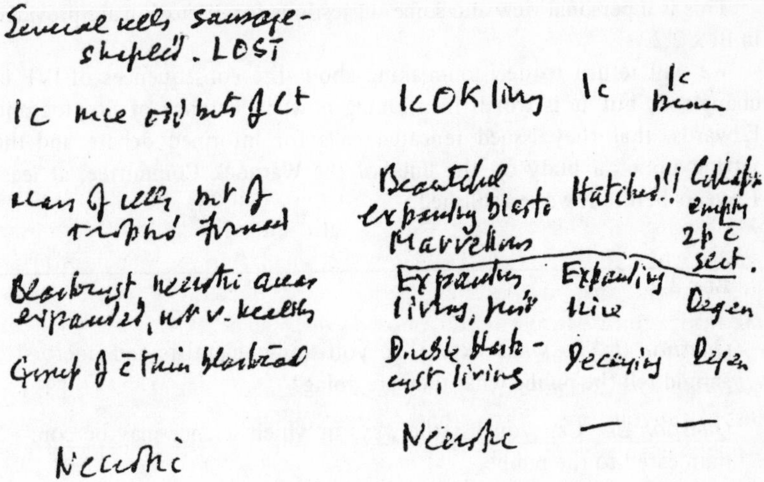

Figure 2.1 *Laboratory notes of R. G. Edwards, showing his reaction to some of the data obtained*

ceptives, and of methods to diagnose genetic diseases. There are also likely to be considerable benefits in the breeding of farm animals and species threatened with extinction. Science is powerful and successful. It works. However its power has lulled some into a position of naive optimism that science can solve all our problems. It cannot. This faith is very strong in medicine, where cancer, heart disease and nervous disorders will all, it is said, yield to science. They may, but it will take time and the answers will not be simple, because these are conditions with many causes and components, which are not all amenable to scientific analysis. Naive faith in science is even more misplaced when applied to world problems such as those of food and population. These are multidisciplinary problems, the solutions to which are complex.

The dilemmas posed by IVF are discussed in chapter 5. Here we may ask what the role of the scientists and doctors should be? Since they developed IVF, does this make them responsible for its consequences? The answer must be no. Society as a whole must bear the responsibility, because, as we have seen, society is inextricably bound up with science. Scientists have a responsibility to communicate what they are doing to the public, to present the state of the art in their field of research and to draw the public's attention to its consequences, wherever this is possible, but beyond this, they should have no more say in the decisions taken about their work than anyone else.

35

This is a personal view and some suggestions for discussion are provided in Box 2.2.

We will return to decision-making about the consequences of IVF in chapter 5, but it is worth mentioning now, in defence of Steptoe and Edwards, that they issued repeated calls for informed debate and the setting up of a body on the lines of the Warnock Committee, at least 12 years before it was established.

Box 2.2

Question 1: To what extent do you think scientists and doctors should tell the public what they are doing?

Question 2a: Can you list the ways in which science may be communicated to the public.

      2b: How effective are these channels of communication?

Question 3: If you had played a part in the development of IVF
(a) how responsible would you feel for the effect of your work on society?
(b) what would you wish to do about it?

---

(12) It is a sterile society which says: 'We know enough, why search for more?'

Some of those who object to IVF and particularly to research on human embryos argue that since the treatment is established, there is no need for further research. They ignore the facts that IVF could not have been established without research, that success rates are low and that research is needed to improve them. But there is a deeper reason why responsible research should continue; this has been well-described by the Rev. Prof. Dunstan, a moral theologian. He has said:

"We know enough, why search for more is a lurking, insidious threat to creative humanity ... Humility is proper to science. One feature of humility is to recognise how much yet remains to be learned, how much good yet to be done. Disciplined curiosity is part of the nature with which humankind is endowed."

3   Infertility

One of the unexpected benefits of IVF is that it has focused attention on the general problem of human infertility. Until recently, infertile couples were likely to have considered themselves as inadequate and as failures. Many will have been stigmatised by parents, relatives, friends and much of society, and as a result, made to feel guilty, when in fact they were blameless. Robert Winston, a distinguished gynaecologist at the Hammersmith Hospital in London in a splendid, reassuring book called *Infertility; a sympathetic approach*, has documented the feelings of those who find they are infertile. They range from disbelief, anger and frustration to depression, grief and bereavement. Edwards and Steptoe in their book *A Matter of Life* continually point to their great desire to do something to alleviate the feelings of helplessness experienced by the infertile. Infertility is indeed a distressing condition and an illness that needs to be treated.

This is seen even more to be the case when it is realised how many couples are in need of treatment. Estimates of the proportion of infertile marriages have been creeping up in recent years from about 1 in 10 or 12 to as high as 1 in 5 or 6. One reason for this is that couples nowadays are more prepared to admit they are having difficulty. If infertility is defined as the inability to become pregnant after one year of regular unprotected intercourse, then recent data from France has indicated that 1 in 5 couples may be affected. Since there are approximately 350,000 marriages each year in France, this implies 65,000 couples in any one year with problems. A survey of people living in the Bristol area in the U.K. gave a figure of 1 in 6 couples needing specialist help.

As well as being considered more sympathetically, there is a further aspect to the modern view of infertility, namely the recognition that men can be infertile as well as women. That this need be stated so blandly is a commentary on the attitude of many husbands that infertility was automatically their wife's fault. Some men are still reluctant to consider the problem could lie with them, since such an admission has overtones of impotence and a diminished machismo. Even today, the wife may well go on her own to the infertility clinic, although most clinics will not treat her unless the husband attends for full investigation.

In one-third to one-half of cases of infertility, the problem is with the woman, in about one-third with the man, with the remainder being due either to a combination of the two or to some unexplained cause. Doctors, who like to give names to things they do not understand, call this last category 'idiopathic infertility'.

FEMALE INFERTILITY

Female infertility may be grouped under four headings depending on whether the problem is with the ovary, Fallopian tubes, uterine lining or cervical mucus.

(1) Ovulation Problems

When the woman is responsible for the infertility, the problem in about half of them is a failure of ovulation. Over 90 per cent of such cases may be treated successfully with hormones, and it is useful to describe the hormones briefly since they are also used in IVF programmes. The main ones are clomiphene, Human Chorionic Gonadotrophin (HCG), Follicle Stimulating Hormone (FSH), Human Menopausal Gonadotrophin (HMG) and Gonadotrophin Releasing Hormone (GnRH or LHRH).

Clomiphene, known by its trade names, Clomid or Serophene, is very widely prescribed. Although it is not a steroid, its phenolic rings and side chains make it behave as an anti-oestrogen (figure 3.1). The pituitary gland is fooled into thinking that oestrogen levels are low, and responds by releasing FSH which stimulates the ovary.

HCG is similar to luteinising hormone, LH (page 11) and is usually given after clomiphene, just before ovulation is expected.

FSH, known by its trade names, Urofollitrophin or Metrodin, is for those women with an excessively high LH level, but normal FSH. The aim of giving FSH is to adjust the ratio to normal.

HMG, known by its trade name Pergonal, contains a mixture of roughly equal amounts of LH and FSH, and is for those women whose pituitary gland fails to produce sufficient of these hormones.

GnRH or LHRH is for those women in whom there is inadequate stimulation from the hypothalamus. Since this hormone is normally released from the hypothalamus in pulses, it is necessary for a woman to have a small pump attached to her upper arm which can deliver a pulse of GnRH every 90 minutes into a vein. The GnRH stimulates the pituitary gland to release LH and FSH.

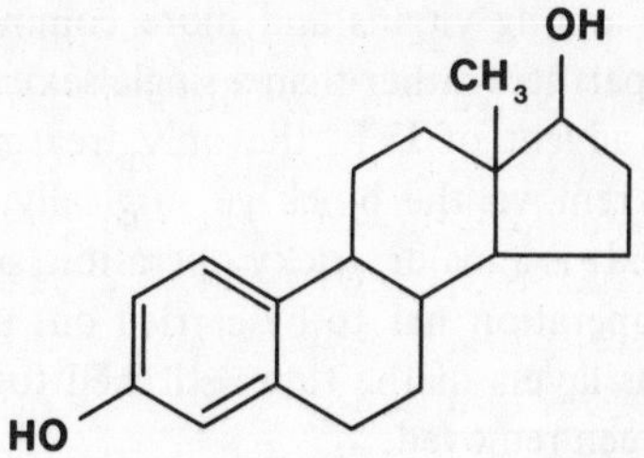

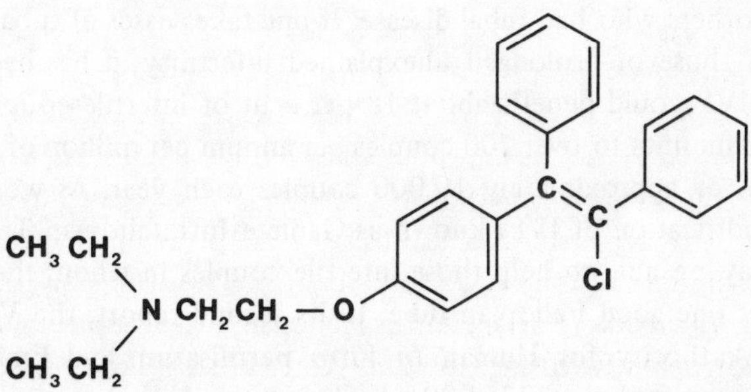

Figure 3.1 *(Upper) Oestradiol 17β, the major biologically active oestrogen. (Lower) Clomiphene*

(2) Fallopian Tube Problems

In about one-third of cases, female infertility is due to disease or damage of the Fallopian tubes. In many cases, one or usually both tubes are completely blocked, so that there is no passage for eggs, sperm or embryos between the ovary and the uterus. In other cases, there may be partial blockage, damage to the mucosal lining or to the muscle wall, or so-called adhesions; strands of tissue which grow from diseased areas and keep the tubes fixed and unable to move, to pick up an egg, for example.

There is uncertainty as to why human tubes become damaged. Much of the damage is thought to follow infection (salpingitis) which leads to inflammation known as pelvic inflammatory disease. Some people imagine that the permissive society and an increase in sexual freedom leading to venereal disease is to blame. This is unfair, though it is true that tubal

39

disease is rare among virgins and more common in those who have had several sexual partners rather than a single sexual partner.

Before the advent of IVF, the only treatment for blocked Fallopian tubes was to remove the blockage surgically. The operation is called a *salpingostomy*. It is a major, tricky operation, since the tubes are small and delicate, the operation has to be carried out under a special microscope, and the various layers of the tubes stitched together one by one after the blockage has been removed.

Depending on how severe is the damage, the average success rate of the operation in terms of a successful pregnancy is about 25 per cent. For those whose infertility results from tubal disease which has not responded to surgery, or for whom surgery was not available, the only answer is IVF. In an analysis of the first 500 births from their IVF clinic at Bourn Hall, Steptoe and Edwards reported that 58 per cent of the babies had been born to mothers who had tubal disease. If one takes cases of tubal damage along with those of prolonged unexplained infertility, it has been calculated that IVF could benefit about 18 per cent of infertile couples in the U.K. This amounts to over 200 couples per annum per million of the total population, or approximately 10,000 couples each year. As we shall see later, a modification of IVF, known as Gamete Intrafallopian Transfer or 'GIFT', may be able to help those infertile couples in whom the woman has at least one good Fallopian tube. In its second report, the Voluntary Licensing Authority for Human *In Vitro* Fertilisation and Embryology (page 75) suggested that 275,000 couples in the U.K. between the ages of 24 and 35 could benefit from IVF and GIFT.

(3) Endometriosis

In this condition, the lining of the uterus, the endometrium, grows in other 'ectopic' sites, typically the ovaries and the ligaments to the uterus itself. It may be the cause of infertility in about 6 per cent of couples. This ectopic endometrium responds to hormones and is shed each month at menstruation. However, it has nowhere to go and accumulates as blood-filled islands of endometrium, which are best removed by surgery. The success rate of the operation in terms of subsequent pregnancy is about 60 per cent.

(4) Mucus Problems

Problems with cervical mucus account for about 5 per cent of female infertility. Mucus is discussed in the next section.

MALE INFERTILITY

As we have seen, male infertility accounts for up to 40 per cent of all cases. In over 90 per cent of these, the problem is that the semen contains too few sperm (oligospermia) or sperm of poor quality or motility. Indeed, sperm defects are the largest single cause of infertility. Cases of azoospermia (no sperm production) occur in less than 5 per cent of males.

If male infertility is suspected, the man will be asked to provide a semen sample for analysis. A normal sample will have a volume of 1.5–6 cm^3, a sperm concentration greater than 20–30 million/cm^3, and 60 per cent of the sperm will be motile and normal-looking. If any of these parameters are not met, it does not necessarily mean that anything is wrong, since abnormal sperm tests are not uncommon. Repeated values below normal indicate that further tests are required. These include testing the ability of sperm to swim (page 19), and the so-called 'post-coital test'. In this, the couple are asked to have intercourse about 8 hours or more before the expected time of ovulation (probably based on temperature charts, though preferably on LH monitoring). The woman then comes to the clinic where the doctor takes a sample of mucus from her cervix, rather in the way it would be done for a cervical smear test. A normal post-coital test would show flowing, stretchable mucus containing live, normal-looking sperm swimming purposefully across the microscope slide. A negative test would show dead sperm, or sperm only moving on the spot. This does not necessarily mean that a couple are infertile, since negative tests are very common in partners with normal fertility. Repeatedly negative tests could indicate a number of possibilities: for example, that the woman's mucus is hostile to the sperm, that she may not be ovulating, that her cervix may be infected or that the man's sperm are indeed abnormal.

A detailed account of the causes of male infertility, its diagnosis and treatment is beyond the scope of this book. Those interested should read Dr Winston's excellent account referred to earlier. Suffice to say that the reasons for low sperm counts and for abnormal sperm are largely unknown and the prognosis for male infertility is generally poor. Only 20 per cent of infertile couples in whom the male is responsible will become pregnant.

Artificial Insemination by Husband (AIH) which is discussed on page 62 is appropriate in only a very small number of cases, and IVF may increasingly become of value for those couples in whom the man's sperm count is on the low side. GIFT may also be an appropriate treatment in these cases.

CONCLUSION

It is important to correct the false impression, often portrayed by the news media, that IVF is a solution for the majority of infertile couples. It is not. IVF is a treatment of last resort. It should only be used after proper tests of a couple's infertility have been carried out, and even then its success rate is low. However, over a thousand test-tube babies have been born following IVF at Bourn Hall Clinic alone, and many thousands of couples stand to benefit from this treatment in the future. The processes involved in IVF are described in the next chapter.

4 IVF in Practice

At the time of writing (early 1988) the number of clinics practising IVF in the U.K. is approaching 40. No two clinics operate in the same manner so that what follows is a general account of the procedures involved. Six stages may be listed (figure 4.1):

1. Ovarian stimulation
2. Egg collection
3. Sperm collection
4. *In vitro* fertilisation
5. Embryo culture
6. Embryo transfer into the uterus.

The Importance of Counselling
Prior to any course of IVF treatment, there must be extensive counselling of the couples involved. In conversations with those involved in such counselling, it emerges that those being counselled are often remarkably well-informed of the procedures involved in IVF and of the likely success rate.

1. OVARIAN STIMULATION

There is a greater chance of pregnancy if more than one embryo is replaced in the uterus. The generation of a number of embryos obviously requires the collection and fertilisation of several oocytes. This is accomplished by giving the woman hormones which stimulate the growth of multiple ovarian follicles. A typical 'hyperstimulation' regime would be to give clomiphene tablets from about the second day of her period, when follicular development begins, until day 6. HMG or FSH injections are given from day 5 until day 10. These hormone treatments stimulate the growth of an average of 7-8 eggs. The next problem is to decide when to collect them. The timing is critical. It is best to collect the eggs shortly before they would

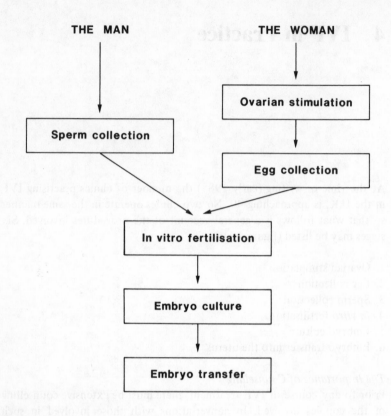

THE MAN   THE WOMAN

Ovarian stimulation

Sperm collection

Egg collection

In vitro fertilisation

Embryo culture

Embryo transfer

Figure 4.1 *The stages of IVF*

normally be ovulated, which, in a typical menstrual cycle, is on the 14th day. This ensures that they are mature and ready to be fertilised.

There are two types of measurements that are used to determine the time for collection.

The first is to monitor the levels of the hormones oestrogen, progesterone and LH in the woman's blood and/or urine. As we saw in chapter 1, the best indicator of when ovulation is imminent is the rise in LH. Chemists' shops now sell kits with which women can monitor their own urinary LH surge and hence predict the best time to have intercourse. The surge has a diurnal variation and most commonly begins early in the morning (figure 4.2). Some IVF clinics monitor the spontaneous LH surge and time egg collection for 28-32 hours after it has started. However, most clinics induce ovulation by giving an injection of HCG, which is identical in its action to LH, and collect the eggs about 36 hours later.

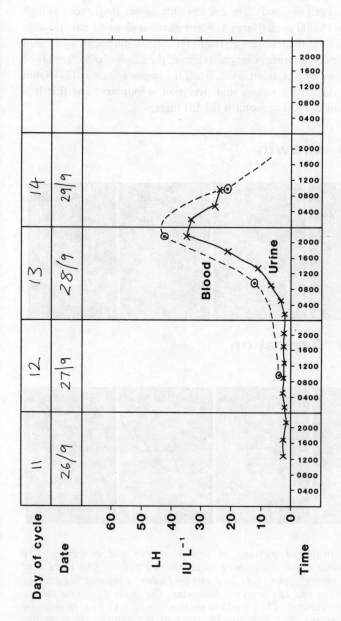

Figure 4.2 The LH surge. (Data courtesy of Dr E. A. Lenton)

45

The second method of monitoring the ovaries uses ultrasound (figure 4.3). This is a form of radiation using sound waves of frequency 1-10 mHz (1-10 million cycles/second). The ear can only detect frequencies as high as 18 kHz or 18,000 cycles/second. When ultrasound waves pass through the body, different tissues cause different reflections and these can be used to form images on a screen. Using ultrasound, the number and diameter of growing follicles may be ascertained. When the largest follicle is 17-18 mm in diameter, the doctor knows that ovulation is imminent and that it is time to administer HCG or monitor the LH surge.

Follicle Growth

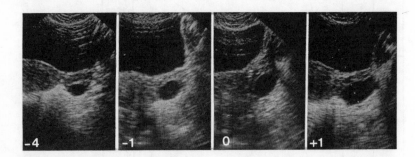

Follicle Aspiration

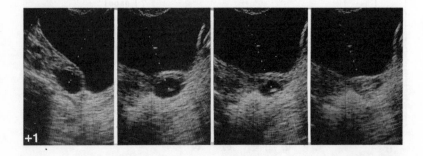

Figure 4.3 *Ultrasound pictures of follicle growth and aspiration. The upper 4 pictures show the growth of an ovarian follicle (the black oval shape in the centre), four (−4), and one (−1) day(s) prior to the peak of the LH surve (0) and one day (+1) following. The lower 4 pictures show a follicle being aspirated. The tip of the suction needle may be seen entering the follicle. As the fluid is aspirated, the follicle collapses. (Photographs courtesy of Dr E. A. Lenton)*

Either way, the aim is to collect the eggs shortly before they are due to be ovulated. This ensures that meiosis will have resumed and that the eggs are virtually ready to be fertilised.

2. EGG COLLECTION

The traditional way of aspirating eggs is by laparoscopy under general anaesthesia (figure 4.4). This is the method which was pioneered by Patrick Steptoe. A thin fibre-optic telescope is inserted into the abdomen through a fine incision near the navel. This enables the surgeon to visualise the ovaries and generally look around inside the abdomen. Laparoscopy is also used to examine the ovaries, Fallopian tubes and uterus to reveal possible causes of infertility. A needle attached to a syringe or suction pump is then introduced into the abdomen through a second, lower incision and the tip guided to the ovary. Each ripe follicle is punctured in turn and its contents withdrawn. The volume of follicular fluid ranges from 2 to 10 cm^3.

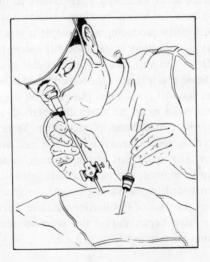

Figure 4.4 *Laparoscopic egg collection. (Courtesy of Serono Laboratories (UK) Ltd*

Ultrasound is increasingly being used instead of the fibre-optic probe to visualise the ovaries. The procedure is simple and need only involve a local anaesthetic. In this case, the doctor introduces the suction needle through the abdomen and then bisects the bladder to reach the ovary, with one eye on the ultrasound screen in order to know exactly where the needle tip is. Another, more recently developed means of reaching the ovaries is to enter via the vagina, and then to puncture the vaginal wall. The ovaries then lie immediately below the site of puncture. Many consider that transvaginal ultrasound-guided follicle aspiration is likely to become the most widely used method for oocyte recovery.

The follicular fluid from each follicle is quickly examined by the embryologist to see whether there is an egg present. If there is, it is removed, together with its cumulus mass, and placed in culture medium for 4-6 hours to complete its maturation and await the arrival of the sperm.

3. SPERM COLLECTION

The man will have been asked not to have intercourse from about day 9 of his wife's cycle so as to ensure a good number of sperm, though some consider this stricture to be unnecessary. He comes to the clinic where a private room is available for him to produce his semen sample by masturbation. If he has difficulty producing a sample, it is arranged for his wife to be with him. It is important to separate the sperm from the seminal plasma since the latter contains factors which inhibit sperm capacitation. The simplest way to do this is to spin the semen fairly slowly and gently in a bench centrifuge, take off the seminal plasma, wash the sperm pellet and repeat the procedure twice more. An alternative method, which may select for more motile sperm, is the 'swim-up' procedure. Typically, 0.5 cm^3 of semen will be carefully placed beneath 2 cm^3 of medium and incubated at $37°C$ for 1 hour. The upper part of the medium, containing the most motile sperm, is then removed, and twice centrifuged and rinsed as above. The sperm are then added to the waiting oocytes to give a concentration of 20-10,000 sperm per cm^3 of fertilisation medium. Sperm capacitation, which will already have begun during the swim-up procedure, is completed in this medium prior to fertilisation itself.

4. *In vitro* FERTILISATION

A variety of media are used for IVF. All contain ions, nutrients and a macromolecule. The composition of a typical medium is given in table 4.1. The ions and their concentrations largely mimic those found in blood plasma. The reasons for including the nutrients were given in chapter 1.

Table 4.1

Constituent	Concentration (mM)
NaCl	99
KCl	1.4
$CaCl_2$	1.8
$MgCl_2.6H_2O$	0.5
$NaHCO_3$	25.0
$Na_2HPO_4.12H_2O$	0.4
Glucose	1.0
Na pyruvate	0.5
Na lactate	5.0
Patient's serum	15 per cent by volume

The medium is equilibrated with a gas mixture containing 5 per cent CO_2 in air. This brings the pH of the medium to about 7.5.

IVF media differ most in their macromolecular content. Most use a small amount of the woman's own serum (that is, the straw-coloured fluid remaining after her blood has been allowed to clot). The main macromolecule in serum is albumin. Some clinics substitute purified human or bovine serum albumin for neat serum.

Successful fertilisation is normally assessed by examining the egg under the microscope, 16–29 hours after inseminsation, and looking for the presence of two pronuclei. Many clinics remove the egg from the sperm and cumulus cells at this time which helps make pronuclei identification easier. In about 10 per cent of cases, three pronuclei are seen. This means, in all probability, that two sperm have entered the egg. Such an egg will divide normally up to about the 8-16 cell stage, and then degenerate.

5. EMBRYO CULTURE

Fertilised eggs are usually cultured for about 48 hours, by which time they will have divided to form a four-cell embryo. Some clinics culture for longer, some for shorter periods of time before transferring the embryos into the uterus. The first test-tube baby, Louise Brown, arose from the transfer of an eight-celled embryo.

6. EMBRYO TRANSFER INTO THE UTERUS

This is a simple, quick procedure. The embryos to be transferred are loaded into a fine plastic tube, which is introduced via the cervix into the potential mother's uterus. In most clinics, this is done without anaesthesia. The embryos are slowly expelled from the tube, and that is that. The woman rests for a while before going home. She will probably be advised to take things easy for a few days.

Pregnancy Testing

There are now reliable, sensitive methods to measure the hormone HCG in blood or urine samples. We will recall that HCG is produced by the embryo during early pregnancy and can be detected as early as 8-10 days after conception. It continues to increase for about 5 weeks, reaching a plateau, and then declines by the end of the first trimester. If HCG rises, it is good evidence that a pregnancy is underway. If HCG does not rise sufficiently, it may indicate that a miscarriage is imminent. An estimated one-third of all IVF pregnancies miscarry. This compares with a figure of 10-15 per cent for those conceived naturally. Higher than average HCG values may indicate a multiple pregnancy.

IVF SUCCESS RATES

It has to be said that IVF success rates leave much to be desired and that we are largely ignorant of the reasons why. A large set of data has been

---

Box 4.1

Success rates of IVF and embryo transfer procedures

(1) Oocytes were successfully recovered from 95 per cent of those women entering an IVF programme.

(2) Of these oocytes, 82 per cent were successfully fertilised.

(3) 24 per cent of the women having embryos transferred became pregnant.

Incidence of pregnancy in relation to number of embryos replaced

No. embryos replaced	Incidence of pregnancy (%)
1	15
2	23
3	31
4	29
All	24

The incidence of aborted pregnancies was 28 per cent which reduced the transfer success rate to about 18 per cent, that is on average no more than 1 in 5 attempts at embryo transfer ended in a successful pregnancy.

If all these figures are taken together, the overall success rate of successful pregnancies per couple entering the IVF programme was 13.5 per cent (that is 95 × 82/100 × 24/100 × 72/100).

Number of single and multiple births

Pregnancies	No. of babies
331 single	331
71 twins	142
9 triplets	27
0 quads	0
411 pregnancies	500 babies

Sex ratio   247 boys : 253 girls.

Incidence of ectopic pregnancy: 2 per cent (compared with 0.3 per cent following conception *in vivo*).

Incidence of abnormalities: there were four abnormalities among the 500 babies. This incidence is similar to that following conception *in vivo*. It is now known that about 25-30 per cent of the embryos conceived by IVF have abnormal chromosomes. Such embryos seem to be rejected by the body, as is also thought to be the case *in vivo*.

published by Steptoe and Edwards on the first 500 births following IVF at their clinic at Bourn Hall, Cambridge. Some features of the data are given in box 4.1.

Two features of the data stand out. The first is the failure of the great majority of embryos to implant. The second is that the success of embryo transfer is increased if more than one embryo is replaced. There has been a great deal of debate among clinicians and others about how many embryos to replace. Most clinics have a limit of three, arguing that to replace more than three increases the risks of multiple pregnancies. The Voluntary Licensing Authority (VLA, page 75) also urges clinics not to exceed three, unless there are exceptional clinical reasons when up to four may be replaced. There is a general feeling that the small chance of triplets, if three embryos are replaced, is acceptable, whereas the risk of quads, quins and even higher-order births if many embryos are replaced, is not. There are a number of reasons for this. To begin with, multiple births are usually born prematurely, with increased risks to the mother and to the survival of the babies. Although most IVF babies are conceived in private clinics, they tend to be born in NHS hospitals. In the case of multiple births, this can impose a severe strain on a hospital's post-natal care facilities. Finally, and crucially, the social effects on a couple of having three, four or more children to look after have also to be considered.

The same problem can arise when fertility drugs are given to women to help them conceive. In some cases, the hormone doses have been misjudged and multiple births have resulted; in one case, in England in August 1987, sextuplets, weighing under 2 pounds each, were delivered prematurely by caesarian section. The public mood of joy at such an event turned to sadness and doubt as the babies struggled but failed to survive. It focused attention on the need to consider not only the rights of couples to have children, but also on the need to consider the circumstances into which a baby will be born.

The criticism levelled at the use of fertility drugs, and the replacement of excessive numbers of embryos following IVF, serves to emphasise the importance of taking a broad view of infertility treatment. This means allowing society as well as doctors to express an opinion, and viewing reproductive technologies as just one aspect of helping couples conceive. It also highlights the need for a statutory body to which these difficult questions could be put. The responses of such a body might not please everybody, but at least the issues will have been raised publicly, and not allowed to proceed by default.

Returning to the biology of IVF, we can see from Box 4.1 that even with three embryos replaced, the success rates after transfer remain low. The problem is that the only means at present available of assessing which embryos to transfer is to examine them under the microscope. This is a poor indicator of their chance of giving rise to a pregnancy, and a better method of assessment is needed.

GAMETE INTRA-FALLOPIAN TRANSFER (GIFT)

GIFT was first reported in 1984 by Dr Ricardo Asch, working in Texas. Instead of fertilisation being carried out *in vitro*, the eggs and sperm are introduced directly into the woman's Fallopian tube. The prerequisite for GIFT is therefore the presence of at least one healthy Fallopian tube. For women whose infertility is due to diseased or missing Fallopian tubes, the only recourse is to IVF. So in what types of infertility could GIFT be of value?

Recent results from Brussels of 100 attempts at GIFT showed that 27 per cent were for endometriosis (page 40), 16 per cent for male infertility and 7 per cent for the presence of antibodies to sperm, in the male or female. 39 per cent were for unexplained infertility and 11 per cent were due to more than one factor.

The GIFT Procedure

The initial stages are similar to those involved in IVF (figures 4.5 and 4.6). Ovarian stimulation is used to obtain several eggs, which are collected by laparoscopy. The sperm are collected by a 'swim-up' procedure (page 48). The most healthy-looking eggs together with 50–100,000 sperm are loaded into a catheter and inserted about 2 cm into the top end of one or both Fallopian tubes. The laparoscopy can be used both to collect the eggs from the ovary and replace them with the sperm into the Fallopian tube. In this way, GIFT avoids the need for *in vitro* fertilisation, embryo culture and embryo transfer. It is therefore not surprising that its success rates are higher than with conventional IVF. Depending on the type of infertility being treated and the number of oocytes replaced, success rates of 25–30 per cent are claimed, and its advocates see it as being of potential benefit to over 50 per cent of infertile couples. While this is most probably being over-optimistic, the procedure does have the virtue that fertilisation and the events which immediately follow it, take place in their natural environment, the Fallopian tube, rather than in a dish, as is the case with IVF.

It is early days for GIFT however, and if the procedure does not work for a given couple, one is not much further on in discovering the reason for their infertility, whereas with IVF, one at least has a good idea whether the eggs, the sperm, the fertilisation process and early embryonic development are functioning normally. Despite these reservations, GIFT obviously has a future. It is a simple, physiological, relatively cheap form of treatment. It reduces the time a woman need be in hospital to a day at the most, and is therefore less stressful to the couple involved.

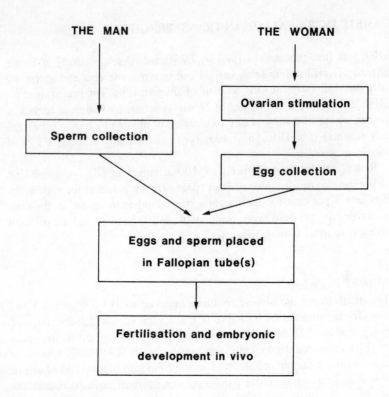

THE MAN

THE WOMAN

Ovarian stimulation

Sperm collection

Egg collection

Eggs and sperm placed
in Fallopian tube(s)

Fertilisation and embryonic
development in vivo

Figure 4.5 *The stages of GIFT*

EGG AND EMBRYO FREEZING

The successful freezing and thawing of mouse embryos was reported independently in 1972, by David Whittingham and Ian Wilmut. However, the first human baby resulting from a frozen and thawed embryo was not born until Boxing Day, 1983, in The Netherlands, and the second, in Australia in the spring of 1984.

The basis of embryo freezing is to allow cooling to take place at a carefully controlled rate in the presence of 'cryoprotective' agents (that is antifreezes) such as glycerol, dimethylsulphoxide, ethylene glycol and propanediol. The aim is to subject the embryos to controlled desiccation, so that they end up looking more like a raisin than a grape, to use an analogy. Once deep-frozen, they may be stored in liquid nitrogen at a temperature of $-196°C$. The evidence to date suggests that they may be stored indefinitely in this condition.

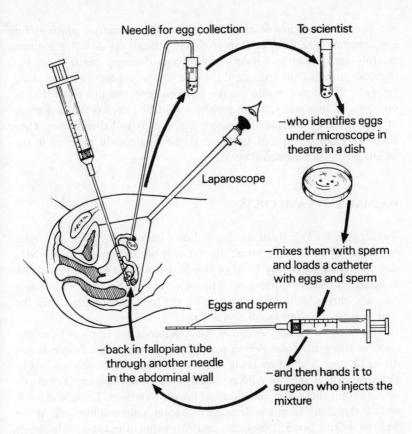

Figure 4.6 *The GIFT procedure. (From Winston, R. M. L.,* Infertility: A Sympathetic Approach, *Martin Dunitz, 1986)*

The first attempts to freeze human embryos were made by Edwards, Steptoe, Whittingham and Jean Purdy, in the mid 1970s. Edwards and Steptoe had realised that there was a particular advantage which might result from the successful cryopreservation of human embryos. If a number of eggs from a patient could be fertilised and the embryos frozen, the woman could wait for a month or two until her hormonal balance had settled down, before an attempt was made to replace the embryos in her uterus. Furthermore, appropriate numbers of embryos could be thawed out each month for successive attempts at embryo transfer, until a pregnancy was achieved.

Pregnancies following the freezing and thawing and subsequent fertilisation of human oocytes, as opposed to embryos, have since been reported.

The significance of this development lies in the possibility it opens up for egg donation (discussed in chapter 5). At present, egg donation requires careful synchronisation between the woman donating her oocytes, the husband providing the sperm and the wife who would receive the resulting embryos. The donor would require a laparoscopy and this could lead to problems of anonymity. These problems would be overcome if a number of eggs could be collected at a single laparoscopy and then frozen. They could be thawed out and fertilised at the appropriate moment in the recipient woman's menstrual cycle.

WAITING LISTS AND COSTS

Waiting lists for IVF treatment depend on whether the clinics are private or run wholly or partially within the National Health Service. For the NHS clinics, waiting times may be anywhere between two and four years, with hundreds of couples queuing up. The majority of IVF clinics are privately run, and this is likely to be the case for the foreseeable future. Here the waiting times are a few months on average.

The National Health Service in the U.K. does not consider infertility treatment in general and IVF in particular as priority areas. People do not die or become disabled by being infertile. Because of this, ready access to IVF treatment is likely to remain private, with the NHS perhaps acting as a safety net for those who cannot afford private treatment. Those who come to IVF clinics are from a wide range of backgrounds and incomes. At the time of writing (early 1988), the cost of treatment in the private clinics is in the range £1000-2500, depending for example, on the way the procedure is carried out, the length of time the patient is in hospital, and the extent to which the NHS contributes to the cost of the hormones used.

One way to bring down the cost of IVF and make it available to more people is to increase its success rate. This will require clinical and basic scientific research, particularly to understand why so few embryos which are replaced in the uterus implant successfully.

Another way of reducing the costs is to reduce the time that the woman spends in hospital. The need for hospitalisation arises largely from the laparoscopy procedure to collect the eggs from the woman's ovary. Laparoscopy is a surgical operation involving a general anaesthetic, and the woman usually has to remain in hospital overnight, returning two days later for the embryo transfer stage.

One way round this problem is being pioneered by researchers at the University Department of Obstetrics and Gynaecology at Sheffield. The key feature of their approach is to dispense with the hyperstimulation regime by which a number of oocytes are induced to ripen, and instead to collect the *single* egg a woman normally ovulates each month. The natural cycle is carefully monitored by measuring LH levels in the blood and urine and when ovulation is imminent, the egg is visualised by ultrasound and collected by a suction needle inserted through the body wall, under local anaesthesia. The procedure can be conducted on an out-patient basis, with less stress and financial outlay to the couple concerned.

During an egg collection being carried out at the Sheffield clinic, the patient was observed to be rather worried about the procedure. However, it turned out to be so quick, simple and painless, that once it was complete and an egg had been spotted in the follicular fluid sample, she said "when are you going to begin?"

The patient goes home for the two days while the fertilised egg is dividing in culture, and then returns briefly to have it replaced in her uterus.

Ethics and IVF

Moral judgements are not absolute, they are negotiable
(Dr Jonathan Miller, 1987)

While IVF has generated a great deal of publicity and comment, such concern over advances in science and medicine is nothing new. Three famous figures who had to contend with opposition to their work, on religious grounds, as has been the case with IVF, are Galileo, Darwin and Freud.

Other areas which have hit the headlines recently include organ transplantation and genetic engineering.

A WAY OF APPROACHING ETHICAL QUESTIONS

It should be emphasised that there can be no 'correct' views of these topics. Everyone has to make up their own minds. All that can be done is to present a variety of views that have already been aired which may help readers make up their minds. This sort of material lends itself well to classroom, seminar or tutorial discussions. As a guide to conducting a discussion, or formal debate, it is useful to consider three levels:

(1) *The individual level* – as illustrated, for example, by the individual or couple being treated by IVF; the sperm donor; the surrogate mother; the research scientist working on human embryos.
(2) *The clinical level* – as illustrated by the doctor(s) and medical staff administering the procedure; the risks involved; the drain on health resources.
(3) *The level of society* – as illustrated by the average citizen; the various pressure groups; governments; politicians.

Each issue requires a balance to be struck between the interests at each level – no easy task.

The issues to be discussed here are as follows:

  (i)   IVF
 (ii)   Sperm, egg and embryo donation
(iii)   Surrogacy
 (iv)   Sex preselection
  (v)   Freezing eggs, sperm and embryos
 (vi)   Cloning
(vii)   Artificial uterus and placenta.

The final topic — Research on human embryos — is the subject of the next chapter.

Before discussing ethics and IVF, it is worth saying a few words about Edwards and Steptoe. Since at least 1971, that is eleven years before the Warnock Committee was established, they made repeated calls for informed debate, committees of enquiry and if needs be, legislation in the emerging field of human embryology. Sadly, their pleas were ignored. Two quotes from a paper in *Nature* by Edwards and Sharpe, illustrate what they were saying in 1971:

> ". . . we believe that it is important at this stage to elaborate the emerging issues in order to give time for defining and evolving social attitudes on which to base rules of conduct for scientists in society. . . to offer comments and suggestions on ways of helping society, science and law to live more safely, harmoniously and with greater confidence in keeping pace with advances in human embryology and other disciplines."

And from the same paper:

> "In human embryology, as in other areas of swift scientific advance, the achievements of science catch unprepared society that lacks either ready-made attitudes or institutional means of forming new ones . . . When scientists clearly foresee potential conflicts with existing rules of society arising from their work, paradoxically both human progress and scientific freedom may hang on their activism in arenas generally regarded as social or political. Scientists may have to make disclosures of their work and its consequences that run against their immediate interests; they may have to stir up public opinion, even lobby for law before legislatures, in the hope that the attitudes of society as evidenced in its laws will mature at a rate not too far

behind the transition of scientific discovery into technological achievement."

Since that time, Edwards in particular, has been in the forefront of the ethical debate, bearing more than his fair share of criticism while no doubt, having more than a few quiet chuckles to himself. After all, his persistence and that of Steptoe, when much of the scientific and medical establishment were against them, resulted in 1978 in the birth of the first baby conceived by IVF.

(i) IVF

Article 12 of *The European Convention on Human Rights* states that "Men and women of marriageable age have the right to marry and found a family." Thus, it can be argued that if some defect in the man or the woman makes the founding of a family impossible, IVF is an acceptable procedure. Phrased in this way, most people would, I think, agree. The objections come in three forms:

(1) There are those who would object on fundamental grounds that it is a deviation from normal procreation, that it is unacceptable to separate procreation from the sexual act. This is a moral, usually religious view that it is impossible to argue against. You either accept it, or you do not.

(2) The second type of counter argument derives from the way IVF is carried out. When it involves superovulation, which is usually the case, more embryos are produced than can be replaced in the uterus. As we have seen, current clinical advice is to replace a maximum of three, or exceptionally four embryos. The remainder may be frozen, discarded or used for research. If all the embryos are replaced, which is contrary to the clinical consensus, at least in the U.K., one is hardly off the moral hook, since not all of them can give rise to pregnancies, and many will die within the uterus. Thus, one way, or another, IVF creates the problem of the 'spare embryos'.

(3) The last type of objection sees IVF as a misuse of resources. Some doctors view it as the one, glamorous end of a cinderella subject — that of infertility treatment, which suffers generally from a lack of funding and status within the NHS. In an ideal world, IVF would be provided, together with the whole gamut of infertility treatments

within the NHS. The reality is different. In the U.K. there are about 10 clinics operating within the NHS alongside over twenty-five private ones.

Recognising widespread public concern about human IVF and embryology, the Government, through the DHSS set up a Committee of Enquiry in July 1982. Its brief was

> "to consider recent and potential developments in medicine and science relating to human fertilisation and embryology; to consider what policies and safeguards should be applied, including consideration of the social, ethical and legal implications of these developments and to make recommendations."

It reported in June 1984. The Committee had sixteen members, seven of whom were women, including the Chairman Dame Mary Warnock, a Philosopher, of Girton College, Cambridge. One member was a non-medical scientist, six were medical doctors, three were legal experts, two were social workers, one the head of a charitable trust, one the chairman of a Health Authority, and one a Professor of Theology.

Not surprisingly, the report had a mixed reception when it appeared since it was never going to please everyone, but is now recognised as an impressive, authoritative, liberal, humane document, which provided a sensible basis for Government legislation.

The Warnock Report is obtainable as a book, *A Question of Life*, which includes two extra chapters by Mary Warnock. It is highly recommended.

The Warnock Committee felt that IVF was an established procedure, that was here to stay. The U.K. government also accepted this principle in its White Paper: *Human Fertilisation and Embryology; A Framework for Legislation* (page 77). The Warnock Committee recommended that a Licensing Body be set up to monitor IVF practice and its consequences, and to consider how best to organise provision within the NHS. They also emphasised the importance of collecting data on the success of the various clinics, so that the public were not misled by over-optimistic claims.

(ii) SPERM, EGG AND EMBRYO DONATION

IVF has led to the possibility of egg donation and embryo donation. The former could assist women unable to produce or ovulate eggs, or who carry a high risk of passing a harmful gene to the embryo; the latter, those couples in whom neither the man nor the woman produced fertile gametes, but in whom the woman had a functioning uterus.

61

(iia) Donor Insemination (also known as Artificial Insemination by Donor, or AID)

Recognising that sperm donation has been available in the U.K. for some time, the Warnock Committee decided to include it within its terms of reference. Artificial insemination by the husband (AIH) was also considered. This is used for example, in cases where the husband is physically disabled and unable to achieve intercourse, or in cases where it is desirable to concentrate the ejaculate and insert it directly into the uterus. It is difficult to see any real objection to AIH.

Sperm and oocyte donation are different matters. It is estimated that at least 2000 babies are born in the U.K. each year following donor insemination. Half the genes of these babies are derived from their true mother, the other half from the donor, who remains anonymous. Most donors in the U.K. are probably medical students.

Although donor insemination is well established, it is not without controversy. The main argument against the practice is that a third person (the semen donor) is introduced into what should be an exclusive relationship between husband and wife. The contrary view is that despite this, for the couple to go to such lengths, the child born following donor insemination is obviously very much wanted.

Strictly speaking, the children born following donor insemination are illegitimate, but in practice, the birth certificate is falsified by inserting the name of the husband rather than the donor, as the true father. The Warnock Committee recommended that the law be changed to allow the husband to be the legally recognised father. This recommendation was subsequently accepted by the Government in its White Paper. It further recommended that there should be no obligation on the part of parents to declare that their baby was conceived following gamete donation. On the question of anonymity, it was felt that the child should eventually have access to limited information about his or her parentage – the ethnic origin and genetic health of the donor, for example – but that a flexible approach be adopted since society's attitude might change in favour of giving more detailed information as in the case of adoption, where the birth certificate may be traced.

(iib) Egg Donation

Egg donation would work as follows. A woman attending a clinic for sterilisation would be asked if she would agree to be superovulated prior to the operation. In this way, a number of ripe oocytes could be recovered from her ovaries, and used as donor eggs. Spare oocytes could also be donated by women undergoing IVF treatment. Whatever their origin, the oocytes could either be fertilised immediately with the sperm of a man

62

whose wife was unable to produce fertile eggs, or frozen for future use. The resulting embryos would be transferred into the infertile wife's uterus.

The baby born of such a union would have half its genes derived from its true father, and half from the woman who donated the eggs. The baby would, of course, be carried for nine months in the womb of its (non-genetic) mother.

It should be emphasised that egg donation is in its infancy. At the time of writing (early 1988) very few babies have been born following such a procedure. Egg donation is obviously much more complicated, as it involves surgery, than donor insemination, and the problem of anonymity is greater. However, if oocyte freezing is perfected, egg donation would become much more straightforward.

In considering attitudes to sperm and egg donation, it is useful to fall back on the individual level and the society level mentioned earlier, and to ask oneself the following questions:

(1) Would I be prepared to allow my eggs or my sperm to be donated?
(2) What would I think of someone who allowed her eggs, or his sperm to be donated?
(3) If I was unable to produce satisfactory eggs or sperm of my own, would I be prepared to accept those from an anonymous donor?

Thinking through the answers to these questions leads, of course, to further questions. Perhaps the most important, if for most of us hypothetical, is:

(4) What would I think when I learned that my mother or my father was not my true genetic parent?

The question is similar to the one faced by those who have been adopted. Those who counsel the adopted and their parents will know that there is no easy answer.

Perhaps the overriding factor to consider is the desperate longing for a child experienced by the childless. Perhaps it is this image that most people would fall back on if asked their views on sperm and egg donation. Suffice to say that most of the submissions to the Warnock Committee were strongly pro sperm donation, and by implication, pro egg donation, since it would be illogical to accept the one and not the other.

(iic) Embryo Donation

This is akin to adoption in that neither the wife nor husband will have contributed to the genetic make-up of the child. The wife though, will have had the experience of carrying the child for nine months. It should be stressed, as with oocyte donation, that the numbers of couples taking advantage of embryo donation is, for the foreseeable future, likely to be very small. The same questions apply as before, though maybe with more force. As the Warnock Committee said, this is "probably the least satisfactory form of donation."

(iii) SURROGACY

Surrogacy occurs when one woman carries a child for another with the intention of handing it over at birth. It has been proposed, for example, for women who do not have a functioning uterus, perhaps because of disease, or in those with a physical disability which makes pregnancy undesirable. There are various forms of surrogacy, depending on the origin of the egg, sperm or embryo. The two most likely are when the husband's sperm is used to inseminate the surrogate mother. This is artificial insemination using the husband's sperm. In this case, half the genes of the offspring will be derived from its true father, half from the surrogate mother. In the other most likely case, the sperm and the eggs will be provided by the husband and wife, fertilised *in vitro*, and transferred into the surrogate mother. In this case, all the genes in the offspring will have been derived from its true parents. The American Fertility Society has suggested that the woman who bears the child be known as a "surrogate gestational mother" in this case. It is worth spelling out this obvious distinction in the genetic make-up in these two cases, because this is precisely what tends not to be done by the news media when they present a surrogate mother story.

Surrogate motherhood is not new:

> "Now Sarai, Abraham's wife bore him no children, and she had a handmaid, an Egyptian, whose name was Hagar. And Sarai said unto Abraham ... I pray thee, go unto my maid, it may be that I (that is, you) may obtain children by her. ... And he went unto Hagar, and she conceived ..." (Genesis 16)

What modern technology allows is for the adulterous aspects of having sexual intercourse with the surrogate mother to be largely overcome by artificial insemination using the husband's sperm, or completely overcome when an embryo resulting from IVF is inserted into the surrogate mother.

Nevertheless, most people probably feel uneasy about surrogacy. Commercialisation has entered the scene, with substantial payments to surrogate mothers. The Warnock Committee recommended that the creation of

64

commercial surrogacy agencies should be a criminal offence, and a bill was passed very quickly by Parliament in the U.K. to this effect.

As with sperm and oocyte donation, it is worth considering surrogacy at the individual level and at the level of society, and asking oneself the following questions:

(1a) If my wife were infertile, would I be prepared to have my sperm impregnate another woman with the object of her bearing the resulting child and handing it over to my wife and myself at birth?

(1b) If I were infertile, would I be prepared to have my husband's sperm impregnate another woman with the object of her bearing the resulting child and handing it over to my husband and myself at birth?

(2a) Would I, as a surrogate mother, be prepared to be impregnated with the semen of a man I did not know, with the object of my carrying the resulting child and handing it over to the man and his wife after birth?

(2b) If so, would I wish to be paid, and if so, how much?

(2c) Would I wish to hand over the child at birth?

(3) What would be my reaction should I discover that I spent the first nine months of my life in the womb of someone who was not my mother?

Perhaps the tone of these questions is unnecessarily loaded against surrogacy. For example, it is possible to imagine two loving sisters, one unable to have a child, the other desperate to help by acting as a surrogate mother. There would be no question of payment in such a case. The child would enter a loving, rather special family. In such a context, free of its commercial aspects, surrogacy may be seen in a different light, a light that some would say should not be extinguished. It is also the case that since the Warnock Committee report was published in 1984, a number of those who were strongly against surrogacy at the time, have softened their attitude.

(iv) SEX PRESELECTION

Of all the developments being considered, this is the most far-reaching, if only because many couples might wish to take advantage of it. For this reason alone, it should be more widely discussed.

The first method for which success is regularly being claimed, and which, if it works, could influence vast numbers of people, is the separation of the two types of sperm, the X and the Y, which are known to differ slightly in mass. This difference is exploited by centrifuging the sperm through viscous solutions to achieve a separation of the two types.

The second method would involve devising a means for determining the sex of an embryo conceived by IVF prior to transferring it into the mother. It is virtually certain that such a method will be developed. Its use would probably be confined initially to those couples at risk of conceiving a child with a sex-linked genetic disorder such as haemophilia, which almost always occurs in boys.

Sex preselection, usually in favour of boys, is already practised in some societies. The methods range from female infanticide to amniocentesis with selective abortion of a female conceptus, the latter being rumoured to occur in the U.K. as well as overseas. Such preselection seems utterly repugnant to many people. It exists because men have traditionally ruled the world and sons are prized, for all sorts of reasons. A discussion of the preference for sons is beyond the scope of this book. Those interested could start with a radical view by Hoskins and Holmes (1984).

What can one say about sex preselection as might one day be possible by sperm separation or embryo typing?

As with egg and sperm donation, and surrogacy, it is useful to consider the level of the individual and to ask oneself the following questions:

(1) Would I like to be able to choose the sex of my children?
(2) If so, would I want to choose the sex of my first child, second child, or subsequent children?

Irrespective of what people may think about sex preselection, development of the techniques for application to domestic species such as cattle, sheep and pigs is going ahead rapidly. There are enormous economic implications in being able to choose the sex of these farm animals.

(v) FREEZING EGGS, SPERM AND EMBRYOS

Some of the background to the techniques for freezing gametes and embryos was given in chapter 4. Frozen human sperm are already used for artificial insemination and present few problems not already considered under sperm donation. Techniques for freezing human eggs and embryos are still being developed, and their success rate is very low. The main question which arises is for how long sperm, eggs and embryos should be cryopreserved, and what should happen to them if the donor(s) dies. The

Warnock Committee proposed a variety of sensible solutions based on the notion of a 'storage authority' to whom responsibility for frozen gametes or embryos would devolve if their owner(s) died. On the question of how long such material should be kept frozen, they recommended reviews of all material held at five-yearly intervals, with a maximum period of ten years in cold storage. In their White Paper on *Human Fertilisation and Embryology* (page 77), the U.K. Government proposed that embryos be stored for a maximum of five years, sperm or eggs for a maximum of ten years.

(vi) CLONING

Identical twins arise in humans by division of the early embryo into two. Each half goes on to form a separate individual in which the genes are identical. This is cloning, albeit on a small scale. In theory, human embryos could be bisected in the laboratory and the two halves transferred into the uterus. Whether couples would wish to have identical twins in this manner is difficult to know. It seems unlikely.

Of more general concern among the public is the production of large numbers of clones from an existing adult(s). The spectre of carbon copies of some Hitlerite figure or Orwellian robot is raised. The copies would be made by removing the nucleus from a fertilised egg and replacing it with a different nucleus from a cell of the egomaniac who wanted himself or herself or some human robot cloned. The procedure has yet to be carried out in mammals and any notion that it is just around the corner for humans is false. We are in danger of entering the realm of science fiction.

Public concern is understandable, however, and the Government White Paper proposed that such practices be made illegal.

(vii) ARTIFICIAL UTERUS AND PLACENTA

Could babies be grown for nine months *in vitro* raising the Orwellian spectre of glass wombs and embryo farms? Short answers are: not in the foreseeable future, and posibly never. However, to allay the public's fears, the Government White Paper proposed that any attempt at such 'ectogenesis' be a criminal offence.

6 Research on Human Embryos

This is the topic over which there has been the most controversy and the one in which the many aspects of IVF – biological, medical, social and ethical – are brought together. Some people feel very very strongly about this issue. They are passionately, even fanatically against research on human embryos. We will come to their views shortly.

To begin with, it is useful to remind ourselves of the biological entity we are considering (figure 6.1). The fertilised human egg stays for about three days in the oviduct and divides into two, four, eight and sixteen cells forming a morula. At this stage it enters the uterus and changes into a blastocyst which resides in the lumen of the womb for two or three days before beginning to implant in the wall. Implantation begins on day 6 or 7 and is thought to be complete by about day 12.

On day 15, an event of some significance occurs, namely the formation of the so-called primitive streak. This is a groove which marks the beginning of the individual development of the embryo, since at any point up to this time, twins can be formed by the embryo dividing into two. Beyond day 15, it is committed, if it survives, to becoming a single individual. Outside the uterus, in a culture dish for example, the early embryo will not survive more than a few days.

We can see how these biological events had an influence on the time limit for research on human embryos suggested by the Warnock committee. They chose 14 days, that is before the primitive streak begins to form. The Government, in its White Paper, also chose 14 days or the appearance of the primitive streak, whichever was sooner, as the cut-off point if research were to be permitted.

Many of the general public may well think that a 14-day human embryo has a head, a body, arms and legs but rest assured, it does not! The 14-day human embryo is a tiny blob of cells about the size of a full stop. Even at three weeks it is no bigger than a grain of rice. The fully-fledged nervous system and any notions of consciousness are many weeks off. The human embryo does not become recognisably human until the sixth to seventh week of pregnancy.

68

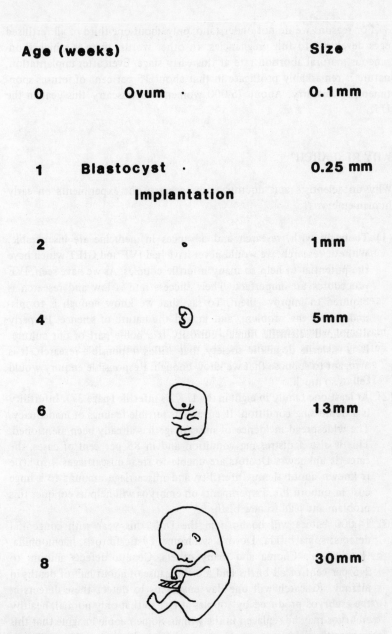

Age (weeks)		Size
0	Ovum ·	0.1mm
1	Blastocyst ·	0.25 mm
	Implantation	
2		1mm
4		5mm
6		13mm
8		30mm

Figure 6.1 *Life size diagram of the early stages of human development. 'Size' refers to diameter or length, as appropriate*

For reasons we do not understand, only about one-third of all fertilised eggs develop into full pregnancies. In other words, there is a high spontaneous, natural abortion rate at this early stage. Even after implantation, nature is remarkably profligate in that about 15 per cent of fetuses spontaneously miscarry. About 75,000 women will miscarry this year in the U.K.

WHY RESEARCH?

Why do scientists and doctors wish to carry out experiments on early human embryos?

(1) To begin with, research and advances in medicine are inseparable. Without research, we would never have had IVF and GIFT which have the potential to help so many infertile couples. As we have seen, IVF procedures are imperfect. Their success rate is low and research is required to improve them. To say that we know enough is to misunderstand the problem, and indeed the nature of science. Properly disciplined scientific human curiosity is a noble part of our culture. It is a sterile dogmatic society that stifles responsible research. It is arrogant to suppose that we know enough. Responsible enquiry would tell us so much.

(2) At least one family in eight in the U.K. is infertile (page 37). Infertility is a depressing condition. It engenders terrible feelings of inadequacy. The widespread incidence of miscarriage has already been mentioned. This is also a distressing condition and in 85 per cent of cases, the cause is unknown. Doctors are unable to treat miscarriages – so little is known about them. Infertility and miscarriage amount to a huge cost in unborn life. Experiments on embryos will help us conquer this problem and lead to new births.

(3) 14,000 babies will be born in the U.K. this year with congenital defects; spina bifida, Down's syndrome, cystic fibrosis, haemophilia, Huntington's Chorea and many others. Genetic defects amount to 2–5 per cent of all births and are the cause of about half of deaths in infancy. Research will one day enable us to detect these defects in the embryos produced by couples at risk so that only normal, healthy embryos may be replaced in the womb. Some people imagine that this implies the deliberate genetic manipulation of human embryos. This is not the case. In a group of embryos from couples at risk, some will be normal, some abnormal. Research will offer us the possibility of selecting the normal and assisting in their development to produce healthy babies.

It is true that many genetic defects can be detected later in pregnancy by the technique of amniocentesis of which over 20,000 are carried out annually in the U.K. A needle is inserted under anaesthetic into the amniotic fluid surrounding the fetus. The fluid which is withdrawn contains cells, derived mainly from the amniotic membranes, skin, and digestive, respiratory and urinogenital passages of the fetus. The cells are placed in a suitable medium so that they multiply. When a sufficient number is obtained, they are harvested and tested biochemically for suspected genetic abnormalities. The optimum time for carrying out amniocentesis is the 15th–16th week of pregnancy. The only 'treatment' for a positive diagnosis is for the mother to have an abortion. The same is true for a more recent technique, that of chorion biopsy in which embryonic tissue may be obtained between 8 and 12 weeks of pregnancy. Ultrasound is used to visualise the fetus, and a small amount of the placental tissue which surrounds it is aspirated, usually by inserting a catheter through the cervix, that is without having to make an incision or needle puncture in the mother's abdomen.

It would obviously be less traumatic if genetic defects could be detected at the preimplantation embryo stage. This would require the embryo to be conceived by IVF, or possibly to be flushed from the uterus at the blastocyst stage following normal intercourse, fertilisation and early development. This latter technique is known as 'lavage'. Either way, the preimplantation embryo(s) would be assessed for a specific genetic or chromosomal defect, and only the healthy one(s) replaced in the uterus.

(4) Many cases of infertility defy diagnosis; about 40,000 couples in the U.K. fall into this category. It would be valuable in many cases to examine the oocytes and sperm, to fertilise them *in vitro*, and see if the embryos develop normally. Research would be required to define what is 'normal' and what is not.

(5) As with research into many aspects of reproduction, benefits can come not only in assisting fertility, but in preventing it, that is in the development of contraceptives. It might be imagined that present contraceptives are adequate. This is far from being the case. The World Health Organization for example, spends about £10m a year on a programme of research, development and research training in human reproduction. They sponsor research on antifertility vaccines, intrauterine devices, post-ovulatory methods (popularly known as 'morning after pills') and methods for the regulation of male fertility, to name but four areas, and some of their projects are likely to warrant the use of human embryos.

(6) Finally, we have the opportunity to observe how one human cell becomes different from its neighbour. This process of differentiation

71

is one of the last biological frontiers. If we understood the mechanism of differentiation, we might understand the origin of cancer, because in one sense, cancer cells are like embryo cells. They divide rapidly and repeatedly. In another sense, they are the opposite of embryo cells in not knowing when to stop. They are embryo cells gone wild. As we have seen in chapter 2, the outcome of research cannot be predicted. If it could, there would be no need to do it, so it would be foolish to say that research on human embryos will definitely lead us to understand cancer. But we come back to the starting point of this section on research; it is a negative society that fails to try.

THE ORIGIN OF HUMAN EMBRYOS USED FOR RESEARCH

Where do human embryos for research come from? They arise in two ways; as 'spare' embryos from IVF programmes and by the fertilisation of donor eggs with donor sperm. The latter are known as 'research embryos'.

When a woman is superovulated prior to IVF in a typical clinic, she produces on average 7–8 ripe eggs. An attempt will be made to fertilise them all and the three 'best' embryos will be transferred into the uterus. The four or five embryos remaining may be cryopreserved for replacement in a subsequent menstrual cycle. If the parents decline to have their embryos frozen or if they appear abnormal, they may be used for research purposes, subject to the approval of the parents, the local ethical committee and in the U.K., the Voluntary Licensing Authority (see page 75). Such embryos have obviously arisen as a by-product of a therapeutic purpose, IVF, and many people would probably be happy for them to be used for research.

The use of embryos made specifically for research purposes has aroused more controversy. They originate as follows: a woman attending a clinic for sterilisation, in which the ovaries are removed, would be asked if she were willing to be superovulated prior to the operation. This would only involve her in having two hormone injections. The operation would be virtually the same. The donated oocytes would be fertilised with donor sperm and the embryos used for research purposes. Much work along these lines was obviously carried out by Edwards and Steptoe prior to the birth of the first 'test-tube' baby in 1978.

Biologically speaking, there is no difference between the 'spare' embryos conceived with IVF in mind, and those made specifically for research purposes, and many scientists and doctors see no moral distinction either.

However, some take the view that human embryos should only be brought into existence with the possibility of their being able to give rise to a pregnancy. Four members of the Warnock Committee took this view and opposed the creation of 'research embryos' while sanctioning research on 'spare' embryos. Three members were totally opposed to any research on human embryos, be they 'spare' or 'research' embryos. This left nine members approving of research, and seeing no distinction between the two types of embryo. The U.K. Government in its White Paper also drew no distinction. It is worth mentioning that a study in Edinburgh indicated that the vast majority of women undergoing sterilisation *were* prepared to donate their eggs for research purposes.

FUNDAMENTAL OBJECTIONS TO RESEARCH ON HUMAN EMBRYOS

Most of those who object passionately to any research on human embryos think, quite simply, that human life begins at fertilisation because the soul enters at this point, and that the human embryo is therefore a small, defenceless human being. Such people use the terms 'human life' and 'human being' and 'human status' to refer equally to a newborn baby, a child, an adult, an old person and an early embryo, indeed anything from the point of conception, which, in practice is post-fertilisation is to them, a fully-fledged human being. No reason is given for this belief. It is something one believes or does not believe. If you do believe this, then research on human embryos is obviously out of the question. Some of the arguments which are used to counter this belief are as follows:

(1) We have seen that many, perhaps two-thirds of all embryos conceived *in vivo*, abort spontaneously. Does this amount to killing human beings? If not, why not?

Do the thousands of women in the U.K. who use the intra-uterine device, which works as a contraceptive by preventing the implantation of the embryo in the uterus, consider they are killing human beings?

(2) As we saw in chapter 1, very few of the hundreds of cells which make up the early embryo will actually develop into the new offspring. Most of the cells at this early stage become part of the membranes around the embryo, such as the placenta. In addition, cells which might have been expected to become part of the fetus may sometimes become something not recognisably human at all, for example, a malignant growth known as the hydatidiform mole. To those who consider the fertilised egg a human being, we can ask why such a high proportion of 'human beings' die before they are even born?

(3) English Common Law does not recognise legal personality, that is, the bearing of rights, until after live birth. The law does not treat the embryo as having a right to life. This is, of course, not to say that because the embryo has no rights in legal terms, it does not exert some moral claim on us. We have a duty to weigh its moral claim in any decision with regard to how we handle it.

The argument that the early human embryo should be afforded the status of a human being conflicts with a moral tradition going back over 2000 years. It was originally expressed in terms of the laws concerning abortion. For example, for many centuries throughout the Christian era, the crucial point was the time around which the fetus quickened in the womb. After this point, it gained a special status. This was taken to be at about 40 days, which happens to coincide with the point when the fetus becomes recognisably human. After this point, a pregnant woman could not be hanged for murder since this would have meant the death of the growing infant. Homicide would also have been feticide. This long established Roman Catholic tradition was only changed by Pope Pius IX in 1869. In other words, it is only since 1869 that Roman Catholics have proffered absolute protection to the human embryo from the moment of conception.

Some who oppose research on human embryos adopt a less extreme position by saying that early human embryos have the potential to become human beings and that research on human embryos is therefore research on potential human beings. Superficially, this might seem a persuasive point of view, but in reality, an early human embryo in a culture dish has no potential on its own to become a human being. It would need to be transferred into a receptive uterus, and once there, as we have seen, its chances of giving rise to a pregnancy are small.

Many might still wonder: when does human life begin?

To some, the question is not meaningful. It is like asking, 'when does a child become an adult?' or 'when does an acorn become an oak tree?'.

Many scientists would say that the question is not meaningful because the events which precede and follow fertilisation are continuous. Eggs are alive and sperm are alive, as are embryos and babies. There is no one point at which human life begins.

If a fertilised egg is not a human being in the sense that most people use the expression 'human being', a new-born baby is undeniably a human being. So is it possible to narrow down the nine months' window of pregnancy and point, if not to a specific time, to a span of time at the end of which there exists a human being? The answer most people would probably give is yes, but then they would give different answers to the span of time involved. Some might say that the fetus has only to be recognisably human, but would people agree on when this was? Others might think less in terms of physical appearance and more in terms of higher levels of consciousness. But would people agree on when 'higher centres' were uniquely human? In other words, to ask the question 'when does human life begin?' does not help very much. It is also worth reiterating that as regards research on human embryos, we should only be considering the embryo until day 14.

THE VOLUNTARY LICENSING AUTHORITY

Realising that the government was unlikely to bring in immediate legislation to control research involving IVF, the Medical Research Council (MRC) and the Royal College of Obstetricians and Gynaecologists (RCOG) set up a 'Voluntary Licensing Authority' (VLA) under which work could be carried out. The setting up of such a body was also recommended by the Warnock Committee. The MRC funds about half of the medical research in the U.K., including some on human embryos, while the RCOG is the obvious body to oversee the clinical aspects of IVF.

The VLA has fourteen members. In common with the Warnock Committee, the chairman is a woman and a lay person, Dame Mary Donaldson, who was once Lord Mayor of London. While its medical contingent is strong, so is its lay contingent.

The VLA drew up guidelines for both the clinical and research applications of human IVF.

In the light of these guidelines, clinical and scientific centres engaged on research on IVF were invited to submit their research proposals to the VLA.

Each laboratory so-doing was visited, and if its proposals were found to be satisfactory on scientific and ethical grounds, granted a licence to proceed with the work. It should be added that ethical approval would invariably be contingent on the approval of local ethical committees and the consent of the patients.

Throughout its guidelines, and its first report, the VLA used the expression 'pre-embryo' instead of the more traditional 'embryo'. This is because on strict zoological grounds, the 'embryo' is defined as the stage of development at which the primitive streak appears, around day 15 (page 68), and after which there is the certainty that an embryo is committed to becoming a single individual, a twin, or perhaps an abnormal form such as a hydatidiform mole. They termed the embryo prior to this stage, the 'pre-embryo'.

75

It has to be said that there has been little enthusiasm for this terminology among clinicians and scientists. It has been described as playing with words and confusing the public who must have enough trouble already with the jargon in this field. It leads to mouthfuls like 'preimplantation pre-embryo'. Worst, it has given the opponents of research on human embryos the chance to claim the public are being deceived. The term 'pre-embryo' might just catch on but the Government did not use it in its White Paper.

7 The Response of Government

Following publication of the Warnock Report in June 1984, the U.K. Government, through the Department of Health and Social Security, produced a Consultation Paper in December 1986: *Legislation on Human Infertility Services and Embryo Research*. The Government had indicated that it intended to introduce legislation, and the aim of the Consultation Paper was to allow interested organisations and the public to comment on their proposals. The Paper was essentially a summary of the Warnock Committee proposals, together with some background information. Since the whole issue of human infertility and embryo research is very much for the individual conscience and transcends party political differences, the Paper did not attempt to be dogmatic, but to frame its proposals as alternatives, options and requests for clarification and guidance. Those who wished to comment were allowed six months to do so.

The Government then published a full White Paper in November 1987 entitled *Human Fertilisation and Embryology: A Framework for Legislation*.

Its main feature, in agreement with the Warnock Committee Recommendations, was a proposal to establish an independent Statutory Licensing Authority (SLA), very much on the lines of the VLA, with strong lay representation (at least half its members). The brief of the SLA would be

"to regulate and monitor practice in relation to those sensitive areas which raise fundamental ethical questions."

In other words, while the Government accepted that IVF had become a reality and could not be disinvented, the SLA, like the VLA, would go beyond questions relating to the purely clinical aspects of IVF, and consider the wider ethical issues. This would mean overseeing the following areas:

- any research or treatment involving human embryos created *in vitro*, or procured from the womb of a woman (for example, by lavage)

- treatments involving the use of donated gametes (such as AID) or donated embryos
- the storage, in an arrested state of development, of human gametes or embryos for use at a later date (that is, freezing techniques)
- the use of diagnostic tests which involved the penetration by human sperm of an animal ovum

Translated into actual practice, the SLA would have the following functions:

- to license those providing infertility services involving treatment techniques such as IVF, AID and egg/embryo donation
- to license the storage of human embryos and gametes
- to license the diagnostic use of techniques involving the penetration of a non-human ovum by human sperm
- to license research projects involving the use of human embryos
- to advise Ministers on medical and scientific developments in the fields of infertility and human embryo research
- to collect data on the facilities for infertility treatment under its control, and on research currently in progress using human gametes or embryos
- to provide guidance on good practice in the areas for which it was responsible
- to maintain a register of information about gamete/embryo donors which would be accessible to children born of donor gamete/embryo techniques

Without an appropriate licence from the SLA, it would be a criminal offence:

(1) to bring into existence, use or store a human embryo outside the body, and
(2) to use donated gametes to create, by artificial means, an embryo inside the body (that is, using techniques such as GIFT or AID).

HUMAN EMBRYO RESEARCH

This was expected to be the most controversial area, and as in the Consultation Paper, the White Paper included alternative sets of clauses on human embryo research, on which Members of Parliament would be allowed a free vote. In the words of the White Paper:

> ". . . references to the SLA's role in research on human embryos have been included to make clear what the position would be should Parliament decide to permit such research on a limited basis. Their presence does not, of course, in any way seek to pre-empt that decision, and the references have therefore been placed in square brackets."

The White Paper accepted the Warnock Committee recommendation, that should research be permitted:

> "the authority will not be able to give a licence for the use of embryos beyond fourteen days, or after the appearance of the primitive streak, whichever is the earlier. Use beyond this point would therefore be a criminal offence."

However, the White Paper drew a distinction between two types of embryo research: that carried out solely on embryos destined to be replaced in the potential mother, and that carried out on 'spare' embryos, not destined to be replaced. Alternative draft clauses were proposed along the following lines:

(1) "It will be a criminal offence to carry out procedures on a human embryo other than those aimed at preparing the embryo for transfer to the uterus of a woman; or those carried out to ascertain the suitability of that embryo for the intended transfer."

(2) "Except as part of a project specifically licensed by the SLA, it will be a criminal offence to carry out any procedures on a human embryo other than those aimed at preparing the embryo for transfer to the uterus of a woman or those carried out to ascertain the suitability of that embryo for the intended transfer."

To many scientists and doctors, these alternative clauses were a nonsense. It would be quite wrong, indeed, unethical, they said, to carry out research procedures on embryos destined to be replaced in the mother, without first having checked out the safety of the procedures on spare embryos.

If this aspect of research was controversial, other areas of prohibited research in the White Paper were less so.

79

PROHIBITED RESEARCH

To allay public fears, the following three areas of research were prohibited:

- Techniques which would allow the artificial creation of human beings with certain pre-determined characteristics through modification of an early embryo's genetic structure. (The White Paper acknowledged that the technical prospects for achieving this were in fact extremely remote)
- The production artificially of two or more genetically identical individuals by nucleus substitution (that is, cloning). The White Paper again acknowledged that there was no knowledge of such work being carried out artificially with human embryos
- The transfer of a human embryo to the uterus (or any other part) of another species and vice versa and any procedures involving fusion of cells of a human embryo with cells of the embryo of another species (that is, the creation of hybrids)

A possible exception to this last recommendation was the so-called 'hamster test'. In this, the capacity of human sperm for fertilisation is tested by allowing them to penetrate a golden hamster egg from which the zona pellucida has been removed. The White Paper recommended that if the test were permitted, the resulting hybrid embryos not be allowed to proceed beyond the two-cell stage (which they have trouble doing anyway!).

There now follows a summary of the other main proposals in the White Paper, some of which have already been referred to in chapter 5.

THE CONTROL AND STORAGE OF HUMAN GAMETES/EMBRYOS

This topic was discussed in some detail, and the main recommendations in the White Paper were as follows:

- that storage of gametes and embryos by freezing should be permitted under licence from the SLA
- that embryos could be stored for a maximum of 5 years, gametes for a maximum of 10 years
- that embryos and gametes could only be stored with the signed consent of the donors, and could only be used by the licence holder responsible for storage for the purposes specified in that consent (for example, for therapeutic treatment or for research)

- that embryos could not be implanted into another woman, nor used for research, nor destroyed (prior to the expiry of the storage time limit) in the absence of the consent of both donors
- that the sale and purchase of human gametes and embryos should be controlled so as to avoid the risk of commercial exploitation

SURROGACY

The White Paper acknowledged that there was no consensus about the most constructive role that legislation might play in dealing with surrogacy. Views were changing all the time, and while the Government stood by its decision, taken in 1985, to prevent the possible development of commercial surrogacy agencies, it did not feel that further legislation was appropriate.

COUNSELLING

There was agreement on the importance of counselling as a key element in the provision of infertility services. It should enable couples to understand the options available to them such as medical intervention, adoption, and coming to terms with childlessness, and the stresses they might face if they embarked on treatment.

GAMETE AND EMBRYO DONATION

Where treatment using donated material was being considered, counselling should explore the implications for the future parents of having a child which was not genetically their own. Counselling for donors would aim to explain the implications of donation, particularly the legal framework.

On the question of the rights of those born following gamete or embryo donation, which was discussed in chapter 5, the Government's view was that all adults over the age of 18 should have a legal right to find out whether they were born following gamete or embryo donation, and that those who were should have a right of access to certain 'non-identifying' information. In other words, the Government felt that for the present, the donor should remain anonymous. The possibility of granting access to identifying information at some time in the future, was not, however, ruled out.

81

On the question of the legal status of children born following gamete or embryo donation, legislation would make clear that the carrying mother would be regarded in law as the child's mother, and that the donors of the gametes or embryos would have no parental rights or duties in relation to the child. It was proposed that where a woman gave birth to a child following donor insemination, the husband should be required to register as its father, and that the same principle should apply to children born of oocyte or embryo donation.

CONCLUSION

Publication of the White Paper was an event of great historical significance. For the first time, Parliament was to debate scientific issues and experiments which could be a criminal offence.

While the Government were being criticised by some for not coming off the fence on the question of human embryo research, the battle lines were being drawn up, with scientists, clinicians and organisations representing handicapped babies on one side, and pressure groups such as LIFE and The Society for the Protection of the Unborn Child, on the other.

Accounts of the debates on the White Paper in Parliament are given in the last chapter.

8   The Response of Parliament

The House of Commons debate on the White Paper on Human Fertilisation and Embryology took place on 4 February 1988. Prior to this, on 15 January, there had been a discussion on the White Paper in the House of Lords.

THE HOUSE OF LORDS DEBATE ON THE WHITE PAPER

The debate in the Lords, which was of a high standard, was particularly memorable for a contribution by the Archbishop of York. His remarks were widely quoted by the media, and frequently referred to in the subsequent debate in the House of Commons.

The Archbishop, who was himself a scientist before entering the Ministry, generally welcomed the proposals in the White Paper. Like the majority of speakers, he concentrated on the most controversial issue — that of human embryo research.

He said:

". . . that research must continue if *in vitro* fertilisation is to continue. One cannot separate them, and I regard as totally unrealistic and indeed immoral any proposal to continue *in vitro* fertilisation without a proper backing in research.

This is for the simple and basic reason that imperfect techniques without a backing in research are bad practice medically and, I believe, wrong morally. There is a duty to patients to do the best which can be done, and any technique which involves the present traumas and uncertainties and wastage of embryos must be capable of improvement and therefore must be open to research."

He then turned to that most basic of questions, which the Warnock Committee and the White Paper had avoided, but which a theologian had to address:

"What is a fertilised ovum? What are we actually researching on?"

He went over the argument advanced by those who believe that human life and personhood begin at fertilisation; that although there were potential crises for the developing embryo later in its life, fertilisation was the clear, unequivocal point of no-return. He then proceeded to catalogue the difficulties in subscribing to this belief.

"...the uncertainty about which cells are going to develop into the embryo and which into the placenta [implies] a certain fluidity about the identity of the organism at this early stage, and that uncertainty is not resolved until the cells, instead of just going through the process of multiplying as happens in the very early stages, begin differentiating. ... Here it seems to me that one can fix the beginnings of human individuality.

If we are to think of a person in terms of this continuity of history, this beginning of individuality which corresponds in fact with the beginnings of the primitive streak and with the 14 days recommended in the Warnock report, this seems to me a biologically and morally more satisfying starting point than the moment of conception. It is also a way of looking at development which helps to resolve otherwise impossible questions about the human soul.

I do not myself think of the soul as a separate entity, but as the inner reality of a human person. But those who do think of the soul as something infused at a particular moment into a developing organism by God have to face all sorts of conundrums in making sense of it at this early stage.

The other way [of interpreting the status of the early embryo] is in terms of the attributes of personhood. We recognise and value persons in terms of what they are. We see certain qualities and capacities even in a rudimentary form, and the value that we acknowledge in persons implies the recognition of some of these qualities, and in particular the recognition that they are, or can become, subjects of consciousness like ourselves.

Thus on this approach we can see a sort of sliding scale of value in the process of development, and it makes no sense on this view to ascribe full personal value to human matter which possesses none of the attributes which normally belong to persons.

I believe that in the very early stage when personal attributes are non-existent and when identity is yet to be established there is room to allow experiment. But it has to be hedged round by safeguards which make it publicly obvious that respect for our human origins is being properly observed."

The House of Lords debate was also notable for a speech by Baroness Warnock, in which she touched upon the so-called 'slippery slope' argument.

">. . .people often say that if research is permitted using embryos up to 14 days from fertilisation, this length of time will gradually increase. Scientists will come forward to say that if they had a day or two more they could do wonders. Other people say that if we are working on the removal from among us of these very sadly genetically inherited diseases we shall ultimately move on to remove from among us valuable people like myself who are short-sighted.

We can stop our descent down the slippery slope at any point we wish to do so and the way of stopping ourselves descending into unknown horrors is by legislation. If . . . there is the time beyond which embryos may not be legitimately used for research purposes, after which time it will be a criminal offence, then we can stop the descent of the slope at that very point and we shall be seen to do so."

The principal speaker against research on human embryos was the Duke of Norfolk, the leading Roman Catholic layman in the U.K. He said:

"From the moment of its conception — that is fertilisation which includes what is being called at the moment the pre-embryo — I believe that the human embryo becomes a human being. So nothing should be allowed which does not help this human being to live and prosper."

When asked by Lord Morris:

"If life starts at conception, since I am a twin does that mean I only have half a soul?"

the Duke of Norfolk replied:

". . .that is a theological point which the most reverend Primate [that is, the Archbishop of York] has already mentioned. I cannot in any way answer the question. However, I obviously follow the Catholic line, which says that those are vital matters and that it is safer to say that a pre-embryo is the start of human life; a soul is available, so to speak, for the pre-embryo. It is not in my competence to speculate on whether a second soul is available for a twin."

The debate lasted for four and a half hours, and there were over 20 speakers. 17 were broadly in favour of research on human embryos, 4 were firmly against. As Lord Skelmersdale said, summing up for the Government:

". . .your Lordships have pretty well decided the issue today."

THE HOUSE OF COMMONS DEBATE ON THE WHITE PAPER

The debate in this chamber on 4 February 1988 began at 5.45 p.m. and ended at 10.00 p.m.

Prior to the Commons debate, there had been some rowdy exchanges between the Government and the Opposition on the question of the abolition of the Inner London Education Authority. The debate on the White Paper was altogether more civilised. Although there were only 30-40 M.P.s in the House, this was more than made up for by the high quality of their speeches. It was particularly noticeable that far from being scientifically illiterate, a criticism often made of M.P.s, the speeches displayed a deep understanding of the biology of human reproduction and of the ethical issues raised by it.

The debate was opened by the Minister for Health who summarised the key events in the recent history of human fertilisation and embryology: the birth of the first test-tube baby, the Warnock Report, the Government's Consultation document and the White Paper. He said that 70 per cent of respondents to the Consultation document had been in favour of the setting up of a Statutory Licensing Authority, but reiterated the Government's commitment to give M.P.s a free vote on the controversial issues.

There then followed about 20 speeches from M.P.s. The major topic, like that in the House of Lords, was that of research on human embryos, though the composition of the SLA and its accountability to Parliament, the anonymity of sperm donors and the question of NHS funding for infertility treatment were also frequently mentioned.

More speeches were in favour than against allowing research on human embryos, but the majority was nowhere near as clear cut as it had been in the House of Lords. Some of the speeches were very moving, particularly those from M.P.s with direct experience of caring for children with severe genetic disorders. To one such M.P., to ban research on human embryos:

". . .would close the shutters on the faint ray of hope for many families suffering genetic disorders. It would be an act of callous and calculated brutality against thousands of parents and potential parents who have to travel through life with the enormous and depressing responsibility of knowing that their offspring may be afflicted by a crippling condition. Further, those children, even if they are not disabled, have to go through their adult life with the same uncertainty in regard to their offspring."

However, several M.P.s doubted the value of research. As one of them said:

"no-one in the scientific community supporting research has come up with any real evidence to support their claims that the human embryo will provide answers to genetic and congenital diseases, particularly not in respect of experimentation on the human embryo in the first 14 days."

The nub of the argument used by those who objected to research on human embryos was well put by another M.P.

"Those who say that it is not a child point out that the early embryo is a mass of cells, nearly all of which are destined during normal development to form part of the afterbirth. It is morally defensible to give absolute legal protection to this early embryo. From the moment of conception the embryo is a genetically unique, living, individual human being. At conception everything about the new human is established — the colour of hair and eyes, the sex, the eventual height and the complete genetic make-up of the individual with his or her gifts and talents. At conception the human embryo simply has to grow and develop, as at any other stage of life."

How odd, said another Member

"that the Warnock committee was ready to consider treating the human embryo without being clear about what it really was. So odd was it that some members of the committee could not stomach the recommendations to which they were asked to agree. . . .they signed a minority report saying that there should be no experimentation on the human embryo. . ."

Against this, one of the women M.P.s who spoke said:

"We have heard today that one in 10 couples face the problem of infertility. Having gone for treatment, fewer than one in 10 couples go home with babies in their arms. The problem is huge. It is a problem which those of us who are lucky enough to have children will never experience, but we can imagine the inadequacy and emptiness of life when children are very much wanted and are not forthcoming. Who are we to deny those people something that comes so easily to so many of us?

Without a certain amount of research, even those one in 10 mothers would not be taking home their babies. There would be no babies as a result of *in vitro* fertilisation if there had been no research. It is impossible to separate the two."

The M.P. in whose constituency the pioneering work on IVF had been carried out summed up the feelings of many when he said,

". . .the research has created life. . . "

Conclusion

As one of the last M.P.s to speak said, it had been a good debate. It had encompassed, as this book has attempted to do, the biology of fertilisation, the history of IVF, infertility, the clinical practice of IVF, and the ethical issues, above all, that of human embryo research. Did Parliament get its priorities right? It certainly reflected the hopes and concerns of the public. It was now up to the Government to present a full Bill to Parliament. Parliament, on a free vote, was to have the ultimate say, and that, in our democracy, was surely correct.

References and Further Reading

Austin, C. R. and Short, R. G. (eds) *Reproduction in Mammals*, 2nd edn (Cambridge University Press), in 5 volumes:
(1) *Germ cells and fertilization* (1982)
(2) *Embryonic and fetal development* (1982)
(3) *Hormonal control of reproduction* (1984)
(4) *Reproductive fitness* (1984)
(5) *Manipulating reproduction* (1986)
The best series of books in this field. Volume 5 includes a chapter by Cohen, Fehilly and Edwards on 'Alleviating human infertility'.

Barnes, B., *About Science* (Oxford, Blackwell, 1985) pp. 37–71

Beveridge, W. I. B., *Seeds of Discovery* (London, Heinemann Educational Books, 1980)
Very good account of the way scientists go about their work.

Chalmers, A. F., *What is this Thing called Science?* (Milton Keynes, The Open University Press, 1978)
The early chapters are splendid on the nature of science.

CIBA Foundation, *Human Embryo Research: Yes or No?* (London, Tavistock Publications, 1986)
Highly recommended account which includes some interesting dialogue between authorities in this field.

Department of Health and Social Security, *Report of the Committee of Inquiry into Human Fertilisation and Embryology* (London, HMSO, 1984)
This is the Warnock Committee Report.

Edwards, R. G., *Conception in the Human Female* (London, Academic Press, 1980)

Bob Edwards' big black book. A remarkable achievement. All human life is here, in 1087 pages.

Edwards, R. G. and Steptoe, P. C., *A Matter of Life* (London, Hutchinson, 1980)
A very individual account of the events leading to the birth of the world's first test-tube baby.

Findley, A. L. R., *Reproduction and the Fetus* (London, Edward Arnold, 1984)
Strong on the fetal and endocrinological aspects.

Fishel, S. and Symonds, E. M. (eds), *In Vitro Fertilisation: Past: Present: Future* (Oxford, IRL Press, 1986)
A good, substantial account of the many, but largely clinical facets of IVF.

Hoskins, B. B. and Holmes, H. B., in R. Arditti, R. D. Klein and S. Minden (eds), *Test-tube Women* (Pandora Press, London, 1985)

Johnson, M. and Everitt, B., *Essential Reproduction* (Oxford, Blackwell, 1983)
The best medium-sized introduction to this subject.

McLaren, Anne, (1) 'Why study early human development?', *New Scientist*, 24 April 1986, pp. 49-52; (2) 'Can we diagnose genetic disease in pre-embryos?', *New Scientist*, 10 December 1987, pp. 42-47
Two excellent accounts by a highly respected world authority in this area.

Medawar, P. B., *Advice to a Young Scientist* (New York, Harper and Row, 1979)
Recommended for aspiring scientists.

Richards, S., *Philosophy and Sociology of Science: An Introduction* (Oxford, Blackwell, 1983)
The best general introduction to this topic.

Warnock, Mary, *A Question of Life* (Oxford, Blackwell, 1985)
The Warnock Report, with two extra chapters by Mary Warnock

Winston, R. M. L., *Infertility: A Sympathetic Approach* (London, Martin Dunitz, 1986)

Wood, C. and Westmore, A., *Test-tube Conception* (London, Allen and Unwin, 1983)
A distinguished scientist and science journalist provide an Australian perspective.

Index

93